MW00986107

Touch for Health Pocketbook
With Chinese 5 Element Metaphors

Develop Awareness,
Balance Posture and Life Energy,
& Enjoy Your Life

by
John F. Thie, DC
&
Matthew Thie, M.Ed.

An easy, simple, safe system of kinesiology (muscle-testing, and acupressure energy balancing) with **goal-setting** and **creative visualization** to help you:

- **Clarify** your Personal Vision
- **Clear** mental/emotional/ physical and energetic blocks
- **Relieve** pain and release tension
- **& Balance** your energy flow to enhance your personal bests, achieve more consistent and frequent peak performances and reach your life goals

Touch for Health Pocketbook
with Chinese 5 Element Metaphors

Copyright John F. Thie & Matthew Thie 2002

Cover Design: Luther Thie; Layout: MAT

Published by Touch for Health Education
6162 La Gloria Dr.
Malibu, California 90265

ISBN # 0-87516-791-0

A Note from Dr. Thie

I have been working with this system of balancing the energy of the human being for over 30 years now, and I am still amazed how much and how easily it helps people. The potential of people to make shifts in their posture, attitude, and aspirations, whether subtle or dramatic, is a constant source of joy for myself and the people I work with. Now I invite YOU to consider what you really want from life, balance your energy and your muscles for your purposes, relieve your pain and release your tension.

In the mid 1960's George Goodheart, DC, introduced me to the principles of muscle balance, muscle testing and integrating the acupuncture meridian energy system with his method of Applied Kinesiology. Early on I felt that this approach to postural alignment and balance was more than a powerful method for licensed physicians. I saw that the philosophy and many of the simple techniques could easily be learned by lay people to take part in their own health care.

Since that time, the system I developed for my patients, called Touch for Health, has been translated into 23 languages and been taught in at least 100 countries. Athletes have improved their performance. Students have enhanced their learning. Families have alleviated aches and pains and optimized their energy. Doctors and therapists of all kinds have integrated the techniques into their practice and taught their patients to help themselves.

I am so grateful to have these techniques to be able to help people feel better and enjoy their lives more. And I am overwhelmed by the calls and letters and e-mails that I get from all around the world from people who have learned Touch for Health and changed their lives.

A Note from Dr. Thie

This Pocketbook will give you the basic information you need to experience Touch for Health for yourself. For those already familiar with Touch for Health, you may find there is a little bit of new information for you here about Goal-Setting, Muscle Testing, and especially about the Chinese 5 Element Metaphors. This is the first major publication of my complete protocol and instructions for relating these traditional metaphors to our life experience and our imbalances. I hope that your creative exploration of these metaphors contributes to understanding and fulfilling your own purposes and appreciating the meanings of any symptoms.

I know that many people will pick up these ideas and run with them, as so many have already done with the concepts of Touch for Health. Click the links on my website, **www.touch4health.com** and you'll see that this is a field that is expanding in many directions. I also know that there are many who will want personal instruction to "get it right" and get started balancing their energy. I invite you to come spend 5 days with me at Serra Retreat in Malibu and participate in my Intensive Touch for Health workshop in a small group - no more than 10- working directly with me. In 1990 I retired from my chiropractic practice, but I missed helping people. So I have designed my ideal teaching/learning/balancing environment and work intensively with a few people. Check my website listed above for more information. For information and referrals for Certified Touch for Health instructors in North America, log onto **www.tfhka.org** or **www.ikc-info.com** to find the Touch for Health Kinesiology Association in your country.

Whatever your path, I hope this Pocketbook will contribute to your joyful ongoing discovery of your unique talents and missions, and your fulfillment as the unique and precious person that you are.
In Touch,

Dr. John F. Thie,
Malibu, California, March 1, 2002

A Note from Dr. Thie

A Note from Matthew Thie

I grew up with Touch for Health as part of my ordinary experience, pretty much taking it for granted that my dad could fix my aches and pains, and that I could use a few simple reflex points to calm my fears, focus on tasks and regain my equilibrium. Yet I am still amazed by the simple phenomenon of changes in muscle response and the immediate results of energy balancing.

When I do a quick 14-muscle balancing and long-standing pain disappears, never to return, it is a lot of fun. Or when I can teach a friend to help himself relieve pain as it occurs, or improve function over time, it's so satisfying. But what I find most astonishing is when we can transform emotional stress of agonizing problems and challenges into the laughter of new insight, attitudes and possibilities. This is when I realize that it's not just that getting your energy balanced can change your life. The fact is, our energy is always shifting with changing circumstances, and it's natural for our lives to change day by day. But sometimes we hang onto things that aren't what we need anymore, or we get stuck in a fixed posture. When we get an energy balance, all we're doing is facilitating the natural flow of our energies so that we can experience our full range of movement and of emotion.

In its simplest form, Touch for Health involves learning or simply recognizing a few gestures which can clear stress and balance mental energy, allowing greater awareness of what is happening in our life so that we can make clear choices and be more present, effective, and enjoy more whatever we're doing. In its full development it can become an intricate study and exploration of our own personal muscular postures and the inter-relationship of muscles, posture, emotion, energy, attitude and motivation. We facilitate and optimize our ranges of motion, flexibility, function, coordination and strength. We balance the energy of our internal healing or life creating system. We reduce susceptibility to injury or illness, relieve discomfort, and shorten recovery time. Integrating the Chinese 5 Element Metaphors offers a resource for an in-depth exploration of the MEANING(S) of your LIFE-- your hopes, dreams, desires, tasks, duties, goals, passions-- your Vision, AS WELL AS the possible meanings and messages of your symptoms -- pains, fears, inhibitions, stiffness, rigidity, tension.

The most important factor in having success with these techniques is simply whether you do it or not. We are all in the habit of bathing and brushing our teeth. These activities are basic necessities of comfort and well being. We rarely stop to consider that these habits are powerful preventive measures that not only make us feel good today, but keep us from developing all kinds of possible problems. When you develop the habit of balancing your energy, and being aware of what makes your life vibrant and what inhibits your sense of being alive, not only do you enjoy your life now, but you are also preventing untold possible negative developments in the future.

I hope that you will find something in this book that you can adopt as a part of your daily self-care, enhancing present life and your future outlook. If nothing else, (as my dad always says) "Drink more water." But just keep in mind that the biggest challenge to benefiting from these techniques is not learning to monitor muscle response, or to find the reflex points, or master any of the balancing techniques. It is all easy to learn with just a little bit of practice. And that is the only real challenge, putting it into practice. If you decide to try out these techniques, I hope you will find at least one partner who you will practice with on a regular basis. And I hope you will find, as so many have, that your new subtle awareness of your energy is leading you to a more fulfilling life at home and at work, at school and in your community.

Try it, you'll like it!

Matthew Thie,
March 1, 2002, Echo Park, California

A Note from Matthew Thie

CONTENTS

8

CONTENTS

About Touch for Health

When Western chiropractic ideas regarding posture and muscle testing are combined with Eastern energy-flow ideas of chi, or life energy, a new tool becomes available. The vitalistic worldview that the natural human birthright is to be able to use touch to activate their own bodies' natural recuperative powers, or energy, is encompassed by the Touch for Health (TFH) system. These natural recuperative powers are enhanced or inhibited by daily activities. In response to those activities, changes occur within muscles, joints, skin, and all of the organs. The way we feel and function is affected as we become more or less vulnerable to injury and disease according to the balance of our energy. This energy may be called chi, as in the Chinese worldview; ki, from the Japanese; prana, from the Indian; innate intelligence in the Western chiropractic tradition; breath of life, or Ruhah, in the Hebrew and Muslim traditions; Holy Spirit, in the Christian tradition. In each case we refer to the power of the intelligently designed human being to come into harmonious balance as a whole person. In this Pocketbook, we use Soul with a capital S to refer to the integrated totality of the whole person with spiritual, physical, mental and emotional aspects that are not separate from each other, but integrated as a whole.

The Touch for Health system is a model for working with people as whole systems. Our belief is that the physical aspects of the Soul, the whole person, reflect quite accurately the individual energy/communication malfunctions. We believe that a change in any aspect of the person -- mental, emotional, energetic, or physical-- effects all other aspects, since they are all part of the whole person, the Soul. This is physically apparent, though sometimes very subtly and unconsciously. We can often observe postural changes, especially in the facial muscles. We can also observe changes in muscle response as indications of changes in the energy of the Soul.

In the TFH system, we use muscle tests to get a sense of the energy flow in the meridians. We develop goals, assess the flow of energy, use various reflexes to balance energy and then reassess how we feel. Our purpose is to increase awareness of all of the aspects of our whole Soul and to facilitate the flow of energy and communication between all of the cells, organs and organ systems, between the conscious mind, the unconscious, our intuition, and our connection to Chi, life energy, or God.

Our premise is that a sufficient flow of information/energy will result in an emotional, physical, mental and spiritual equilibrium that will allow us to feel whole, to do the things that are most important to us, and to find meaning in life. Creative use of metaphors can enhance our assessment of our own Wellness in the context of our life, help balance our energies towards our goals and help us discover new passions and purposes that are right for us. Awareness is the key aspect of the process. We often feel a lot better physically, mentally and emotionally after a balancing. But the true power of TFH is in developing our awareness of the things that we really want from life and the things that block our energy to accomplish our goals, and empowering us to make choices whole-heartedly for our greatest good.

The **Five Element Metaphors**, the **Organ Function metaphors** and metaphors derived from the **test motions/muscle functions** offer a rich resource for exploring the meanings of our experiences, our feelings, our imbalances and our goals. Using the metaphors helps us to verbalize or at least think about the many possible aspects of our goals and the related imbalances. When we think about a metaphor related to an imbalance indicated by a muscle test, we often have that "Aha!" moment of insight. This may be a highly transcendent, miraculous moment of enlightenment, like those attained in prayer or meditation, or it may also be a step-by-step process of development through small, everyday insights as we deal with our problems, our life's work, and seek our Telos, our life purpose.

About TFH with metaphors

About the Touch for Health Pocketbook with Metaphors

This Pocketbook follows the format of the Touch for Health Reference Folio. It contains quick reference pages to all 14 Meridians, all 42 Muscle-tests, and all of the associated energy-balancing reflex points used in the Touch for Health system. It also contains the first full publication of my creative interpretations of the Chinese 5-Element and Meridian/Organ Metaphors, and metaphors associated with the muscle functions/motions. In order to make the reference pages more useful, and allow this Pocketbook to "stand alone" as an introduction to the Touch for Health system, we have also included some instructions for using the reference pages that are not included in the original Reference Folio as well as explanations of various aspects of Goal Setting and Muscle/Energy balancing.

We suggest that you read through the entire Pocketbook to familiarize yourself with the system before you start practicing the muscle tests and energy balancing. If the muscle tests, or any other aspect of the TFH system is difficult for you to grasp independently, you can refer to the Touch for Health manual, and the Touch for Health video. In addition, the Touch for Health system is taught in four 16-hour modules (TFH I-IV). Certified TFH Instructors have been trained all over the world, and have taught in 102 countries. The TFH Manual has been translated into 23 languages. For an instructor near you, log onto **www.tfhka.org**, in North America or try **www.ikc-info.com** for associations and instructors worldwide. For a schedule of classes taught by the Founder, John F. Thie, DC, check out **www.touch4health.com**, or call 888-796-4568. To order TFH manuals and charts , contact the association, or **www.devorss.com**

Touch for Health involves a model of health and a philosophy of Wellness, which is easy to understand. TFH also involves some manual skills, which require some practice, but can be learned by anyone, either through independent experimentation, or with the help of a Certified TFH Instructor.

KEY TO REFERENCE PAGES

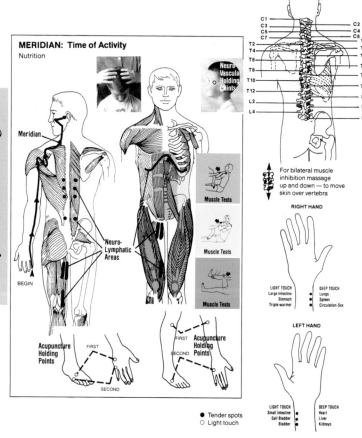

MERIDIAN: Time of Activity
Nutrition

Meridian

BEGIN

Neuro-Lymphatic Areas

Neuro-Vascular Holding Points

Muscle Tests

Muscle Tests

Muscle Tests

Acupuncture Holding Points
FIRST
SECOND

FIRST
SECOND
Acupuncture Holding Points

● Tender spots
○ Light touch

C1
C3
C5
C7
T2
T4
T6
T8
T10
T12
L2
L4

C2
C5
C6
T1
T3
T5
T7
T9
T11
L1
L3
L5

For bilateral muscle inhibition massage up and down — to move skin over vertebra

RIGHT HAND

LIGHT TOUCH
Large Intestine
Stomach
Triple-warmer

DEEP TOUCH
Lungs
Spleen
Circulation-Sex

LEFT HAND

LIGHT TOUCH
Small Intestine
Gall Bladder
Bladder

DEEP TOUCH
Heart
Liver
Kidneys

Key to Reference Pages

KEY to the Reference (chart) Pages

The original Reference Folio was designed as a quick reference tool for those already familiar with the muscle tests and energy-balancing reflex points. It is a flip chart version of the TFH Reference wall chart. These pages now serve as the Reference Pages in this Pocketbook. For those not already familiar with the TFH system, we provide some notes here that will help orient you to TFH in general, as well as guide you in using the reference pages in this Pocketbook.

The "Key to Chart" page shows a general illustration of the elements found on any given Meridian Reference Page. These are the Muscles/Tests and related reflexes of a particular energy pathway or meridian, which is also illustrated on the page.

On the top right of this first page is an illustration of the locations and abbreviations of all of the spinal vertebrae, which is useful in locating the spinal reflex points for bilateral weakness (see next page).

Pulse Points

On the bottom right of this first page are figures of the right and left hands illustrating the "pulse points" which can be used for determining "over-energy". The figure is repeated on the 5-Element Reference Page. To check for over-energy in the meridians, first hold one finger over each of the 3 illustrated points and muscle test, first holding lightly. If there is any indicator muscle change, check each finger individually. The point or points that now cause a change in muscle response indicate over-energy in the meridian. Now check all three holding deeply and re-check individually if there is a change. Do the same on the other wrist, checking light and deep touch.

NOTE: You can also check for over-energy using the **Alarm Points, found on the 24-Hour Law Reference Page**. Check each alarm point by holding 3 fingers over the point and testing an indicator muscle. Bilateral points should be tested on both sides. Indicator change on either side means over-energy in the related meridian.

Meridian Name: Time of Activity
At the top of each chart page is the name of a meridian and the time at which the energy of this meridian is at its highest level. The pathway of this meridian is illustrated on the figure, and all of the muscles and reflex points relate to this meridian. A quick way to balance your energy is to work all of the reflexes for the meridian related to the present time of day. Testing 14 muscles before and after makes it more effective. This is also beneficial for issues that relate to or occur at a specific time of day.

Nutrition
When there is an imbalance in the given meridian, the nutrients listed here may help to balance the energy. (See also: Protocol for balancing with food prior on page 179.)

Spinal Reflex (Bilateral) Points (SR)
Refer to the illustration on the top right hand side of the KEY TO CHART page. This will help you to find the level of each vertebra. Note that the bones provide some landmarks that will make it easier to find a given vertebral level.
The **first Cervical Vertebra (C1)** is at the base of the skull.
C7, at the base of the neck, is the last vertebra that moves with the neck, while T1 will remain stationary,
The first **Thoracic Vertebra(T1)** will usually be the most prominent knob at the base of the neck.
T5 is about midway between the shoulder blades.
T8 or 9 is at the tip of the shoulder blade.
T12, the last Thoracic Vertebra, can be found by following the bottom of the ribcage around to where it attaches to the spine.
The **first Lumber Vertebra (L1)** is just below the end of the ribcage.
L3 is level with the hips.

The spinal reflexes are indicated on the figure on the reference pages as blue or pink vertebra illustrations at the appropriate level. The spinal vertebral levels are abbreviated in the top right hand corner of each colored box containing the Muscle Test Thumbnail Illustrations. The SR is activated by stretching the skin up and down over the center of the spine at the indicated level. The fingers do not slide across the skin, but rather stretch the skin about 1/2 inch up and down. Use these reflexes whenever you find bilateral muscle weakness. Retest both sides and if both sides are strong, move on to the next muscle/meridian. **If one side remains inhibited, work the associated neurolymphatic points**.

Neurolymphatic Massage Points

These points are indicated by dark circles or bands. Use firm massage with the fingertips, searching in the general area indicated for particularly sore spots. Pay particular attention to the sore spots, then retest the muscle. **Challenge** by holding one hand over the reflex points and testing the muscle again. If the muscle becomes inhibited on the challenge, move on to the neurovascular points. If there is any pain in the test range of motion or upon testing, work the neurolymphatics and recheck. A neurolymphatic massage of all of the NL points is beneficial for general soreness etc.

Neurovascular Holding Points

These points are indicated by open circles, usually on the head. They are to be held very lightly, using just enough pressure so that you could slightly tug the skin. Try to feel for distinct pulses on each side and see if they come into sync. Usually 20 or 30 seconds is sufficient, but they may be held longer. **Challenge** by holding one hand over the reflex points and testing the muscle again. If the muscle becomes inhibited on the challenge, move on to tracing the meridian. Since these points are related to balance of the blood flow, particularly in the brain, it is beneficial to activate diverse areas of the brain when using this technique. While holding the points, visualize your desired outcome, focusing on each of the 5 senses in turn. As you shift your attention to different senses, the pulses may go out of sync. and then come back in rhythm after a moment.

About the Reference Pages

Meridian Path Illustration

Tracing the meridian over the body, with an open palm or with the fingertips, will help balance the energy in the meridian and clear any blocks. You do not have to actually touch the person, but try to stay within 3 inches of the body to be most effective. **Challenge** by holding one hand over the beginning or end point of the meridian and testing the muscle again. If the muscle becomes inhibited on the challenge, move on to the reflexes related to the origin/insertion of the muscle.

Muscle Origin/Insertion Illustrations

Sometimes, if a muscle does not seem to respond to the reflex work we are doing, it helps to "wake it up" by simply jiggling the muscle. Refer to the illustration of the muscle, and physically take hold of it with the fingers and wake it up. Pinching in the belly of the muscle will inhibit it, so stretching the belly of the muscle with the fingertips (following the direction of the muscle fibers) will facilitate the muscle. Stretching the muscle away from its attachment points (the origin and insertion points) will facilitate the muscle. Sometimes it is difficult or impossible to work directly upon the belly, or the attachment point of the muscle, yet if you do the reflex as close as possible, it will usually still work. Make sure you let the person know what you are doing and get prior consent before you pinch, stretch or jiggle their muscles. Challenge any of these reflexes by holding one hand over the muscle and testing the muscle (or any indicator muscle) again. If the muscle becomes inhibited on the challenge, move on to the Acupressure Holding Points.

Acupressure Holding Points

These points are indicated by open circles on the limbs. They are to be held very lightly, using just enough pressure so that you could slightly tug the skin. First you hold one pair of points, and then you hold a second pair of points. Challenge by holding one hand over any of the reflex points and testing the muscle again. If working with various reflexes for a given muscle seems to inhibit rather than facilitate the muscle response, there may be over-energy in the meridian. You can use the pulse points or the alarm points to confirm this. Use AHP's "to weaken" which will draw the excess energy into another meridian.

Muscle Test Thumbnail Illustrations
The thumbnail illustrations of the muscle tests are color coded to correspond to the muscle illustrations on the figure. These will give you a basic idea of what the muscle tests look like. The 5 Element Metaphor section provides a text description for each muscle. For more detailed illustrations and descriptions of the muscle tests, refer to the Touch for Health Manual, or your TFH level I-IV Workshops & Workbooks. In the upper left-hand corner of each thumbnail, the corresponding page number in the TFH Manual is provided. The related spinal reflex point is found in the upper right hand corner of each thumbnail

About the Reference Pages

OPTIONS FOR BALANCING
WITH TOUCH FOR HEALTH

1. 14 muscle fix as you go
2. 14 muscle fix as you go, **PLUS** (For each muscle found inhibited, check other muscles for that meridian)
3. 42 muscle fix as you go
4. 14 muscle Assessment with 24 Hour Patterns- Beaver Dam, Triangles, Squares & Spokes
5. 42 muscle Assessment with 24 Hour Patterns
6. 14 or 42 muscle Assessment with 5-Elements Patterns
7. 14/42 muscle Assessment with 5-Element Metaphors
   A. Sound/Emotion Balancing
   B. Color Balancing
   C. Other 5 Element Metaphors
8. 14 or 42 muscle testing and Cross Crawl, followed by any of above.
9. 14 or 42 muscle testing and balance with foods
10. Balancing and then checking for inhibiting foods.
11. Balancing then checking for past, present and/or future emotional stressors (balance with ESR)
12. Visual Inhibition Balancing
13. Auricular Exercise Balancing
14. Figure 8 Balancing
15. Gait Balancing
16. Time of Day Balancing
17. Balancing muscles for a specific malfunction/pain
18. Pain Tapping
19. Pain Relief with Golgi and Spindle Cell reflexes
20. Reactive Muscle Balancing
21. Pain relief by meridian tracing, flushing or massage
22. Simple pain relief by general neurolymphatic massage
23. Pain/impaired function assessment on an analog scale
24. Combinations of techniques
25. Priority testing for best technique (circuit locating)
26. Zip-ups, Switching-On, AIM & Hydration Pre-tests

Options for Balancing with Touch for Health ~ Further Notes
This list of options is meant as a reminder for those who are already familiar with the TFH system. It includes just some of the different techniques in the TFH manual and that are taught in TFH level I-IV Workshops. The following notes are meant to give you an idea of the many applications of TFH, and in some cases, a very basic explanation of how to utilize some of these options. If you want to learn more, refer to your manual, or look into training by a Certified TFH Instructor near you.

Options 1-3: (14, 14+, and 42-Muscle Balancing) **Fix as you go**
The TFH system uses at least one muscle for each of the major meridians (meridians may be thought of as pathways for the "Chi" or life energy). So we test at least 14 muscles- primarily as indicators of the flow of energy in the related meridians. We can then balance the energy in any meridian that we find "blocked" as indicated by a muscle that is inhibited in any way. When we check and balance each meridian, one at a time, we call it "fix as you go". A quick 14-muscle "fix as you go" balance is great as a daily, holistic "tune-up" and can have profound benefits for reaching our specific goals. If we want to be a bit more thorough, we can test 14 muscles PLUS, for each meridian which we find at all "blocked", we can test all the other muscles related to the same meridian. For some meridians, such as the Central, we only have one muscle to test, but others have more. So, for example, if we find an imbalance in the Anterior Serratus, related to the Lung Meridian, we can also test three additional muscles. We can also decide to test all 42 muscle pairs and "fix" (balance) each muscle/meridian we find inhibited. This allows us to be most thorough in assessing, balancing, and reinforcing equilibrium in our energy.

Options 4-7: Assessment Balancing
When we balance energy, we have the option of working the reflexes for each particular imbalance as we find it (fix as you go). We can also test all of the muscles (14, 14+, or 42) and then look at the pattern of

imbalance and choose a logical place to begin balancing. We make an Assessment of all the energy blocks, and then balance. We can look at the patterns in the 24-hour meridian cycle (the Wheel or the Clock) or in the Chinese 5 Element cycles (Shen/Creation cycle and Ko/Control cycle). Often, when we balance a single key meridian, all of the other meridians come into balance (as indicated by all of the related muscles re-testing "strong" or locking in place). Otherwise, we can balance any remaining muscle inhibitions, which will almost always be few.

Options 8-16: Additional "Stand Alone" or "Add-on" Techniques
Each of these additional techniques can be used "stand-alone" to balance our energies, or as an "add-on" technique to help address any residual imbalance after balancing the 14 meridians and getting the energy flowing freely in the whole person. We advocate the holistic 14-meridian approach whenever possible, because this seems to have more profound and lasting results, but any of these can serve as a quick "tune-up" for your energy. For more information on these techniques, refer to the Touch for Health Manual, or your TFH level I-IV Workshops & Workbooks.

Option 17: Balancing Around a Problem Muscle/Area
You can use the "Muscle Diagram" on page 125 in your TFH Manual, or look for related muscles on your reference pages in this Pocketbook, and balance all muscles that might be related to pain or malfunction in a particular muscle or area of the body. Best results are obtained by balancing the 14 meridians first for a positive goal, and then checking muscles related to a problem area. Often, pain or inhibition disappears or is sufficiently reduced without directly addressing the area of pain or dysfunction (This doesn't necessarily mean that physical injuries/conditions have also disappeared, so use common sense and get the appropriate attention).

Options 18-25: More "Stand Alone" or "Add-on" Techniques
Each of these additional techniques can be used "stand-alone" to

balance our energies, or as an "add-on" technique to help address any residual imbalance after balancing the 14 meridians and getting the energy flowing freely in the whole person. We advocate the holistic 14-meridian approach whenever possible, because this seems to have more profound and lasting results, but any of these can serve as a quick "tune-up" for your energy. For more information on these techniques, refer to the Touch for Health Manual, or your TFH level I-IV Workshops & Workbooks.

Option 26: Pre-tests for Relative Hydration, Switching, and AIM
These pre-tests are very helpful for orienting the person helping and the person being balanced. They help develop the mutual sense of energy facilitation and inhibition and also help clear any energetic "scrambling" which might confuse the results of the muscle tests.

Switching On
If we check for "Switching" (electrical scrambling in the body) it is often found when someone is under stress. This would mean that if we started testing and correcting without attending to this "scrambling" we might get less than best results. Especially when we are first learning to muscle test, it is helpful to reduce confusing results due to switching.

For this reason it's a good idea to "switch on" before a balance. We can also switch on any time we feel like we need a little mental clearing, or before we start a challenging task.

How to Switch On
a. Hold the navel with one hand and rub below the collar bone/breast bone junctions(K27, the endpoints of the kidney meridian) with the other hand. Change hands and repeat.
b. Hold the navel and rub just above the center of the upper lips and just below the center of the lower lips (endpoints of Central and Governing Meridians). Change hands and repeat.
c. Hold the navel and rub the tailbone. Change hands and repeat.

Zip-ups

The Central Meridian runs straight up the center of the body. Zipping a finger or the hand from the pubic bone to the lower lip reinforces the normal flow of energy in this major meridian and serves to help clear general energy blocks, especially those related to energy leaving the body. This is another simple thing we can do to for a quick general balancing, and to reduce unexpected results when muscle testing. Trace it 3 times.

PRETESTS

These pretest exercises are very helpful both in clearing extraneous problems, which can confuse our muscle test results, and in orienting ourselves to one another. Especially when we're starting out, it is very helpful to get a clear sense of the difference between a facilitated (locking) muscle and an inhibited (unlocking) muscle.

Accurate Indicator Muscle (AIM) Test

The following are great "first experiments" in muscle testing. We suggest you read the whole muscle testing section and then try these techniques.

(First, "switch on")

1. Check the muscle first

Ask the person to lift their straight arms to about 30° in front of the body. Push down on the arms above the wrists to move them back to the sides of the body. Use less than 2 lbs. (1kg) of pressure for about 2 seconds through 2" (6 cms) , to see if the muscle locks. The arms will either stay firm and "lock", or feel mushy and "unlock". Note, this is the test for the anterior deltoid, see the Gall Bladder Meridian Reference Page for the muscle test thumbnail and reflex points.

2. Correct if not locking

If "mushy", place the fingers of one hand on the Anterior Fontanel of the head while using the other hand to rub the third, fourth and fifth rib spaces beside the breast bone on the front of the chest. The muscle should now lock.

3. Physical Challenge
Introduce a physical stress by manually "turning off" the muscles which are located on the front of the shoulder. Push together in the belly of the muscles and retest. They should now unlock. Stretch apart in the belly of the muscle to facilitate and retest. They should now lock.

4. Unexpected Muscle Response
Sometimes a muscle will not lock/unlock as expected when you check for an Accurate Indicator Muscle. For instance, when testing Anterior Deltoid, pinching or stretching the fibers in the belly of the muscle may not have an effect. The following suggestions may help in this situation. The list is not prioritized.
• Drink some water
• Do some slow, relaxed breathing
• Stimulate the origin and insertion of the muscle
• Check that there is no stress involved (ask)
• Hold E.S.R. points
• Visualize the muscle relaxing or "defrosting"
• Check for recruitment (see muscle testing section)
• Ask the person to be "testable"
• Ask the person to imagine they are pushing the hand into the floor on the arm being tested
• Use your creativity and techniques from the TFH Synthesis.

5. Emotional Challenge
Test the muscles while thinking of something a little bit unpleasant, embarrassing or scary. The muscles should unlock, which is the usual stress response. Have the person think of something pleasant and happy. The muscle should now lock.

6. Biochemical Challenge

If the person were to smell industrial grade ammonia or permanent markers, the muscle will invariably unlock. Even just thinking about rancid grease will have an effect. After breathing fresh air, the indicator muscle should lock when retested.

7. Energetic Challenge

We can incorporate the test for Central Meridian Integrity (see below) as an Energetic Challenge for our AIM test.

After checking our indicator muscle (IM) with the AIM tests, we can use the IM to indicate energy in its related meridian or energy response to different challenges.

Central Meridian Energy

If the energy in the brain is compromised, poor concentration, confusion and vagueness result. This exercise balances the Central Meridian, the energy pathway related to brain function, from the pubic bone to the bottom lip.

Central Meridian Integrity (Zip-Ups) Pre-Test

1. Use a clear circuit indicator muscle.
2. Ask the person to run one hand up their Central Meridian (from pubic bone to bottom lip) and retest IM

Locked = expected response

Unlocked = Central reversal - flush Central Meridian (see below)

3. Have them run one hand down the Central Meridian (opposite direction) and retest IM

Unlocked = usual response

Locked = Over energy in Central- flush Central Meridian (see below)

Meridian Flushing

4. Flush the meridian by brushing your hand up and down several times, ending with two or three traces from pubic bone to bottom lip.

Pretests- Central Meridian

5.   Repeat tests as above after correction. If, after correcting, the problem still exists, ask the person to drop their shoulders and relax, unlock their knees, take a deep breath, "be testable" etc. as in step 4 of AIM test on page 23.

Switching Pre-tests

How Switching Problems Manifest

Side to side switching problems show as confusion between right and left, and the "dyslexic" tendency to confuse "d" and "b".

Top and bottom switching problems show as difficulty walking up and down stairs, disorientation looking down from heights (or looking up), and the dyslexic tendency to confuse "b" and "p".

Front and back switching problems include not being able to reverse a car using the rear vision mirror, and the dyslexic tendency to have handwriting slide up or down as it goes across the page.

1. To clear side to side switching, hold the navel with one hand and rub below the ends of the collarbones (K27's) with the other hand. Switch hands and repeat.

2. To clear top and bottom switching, hold the navel with one hand. Rub the top and bottom lips with the other hand. Switch hands and repeat.

3. To clear front and back switching problems, hold the navel with one hand. Rub the tailbone with the other hand. Switch hands and repeat.

Switching Pretest using Circuit Locating

Before muscle testing, both tester and testee must be switched on. We can use Circuit Locating to be specific about the type of switching involved when we are stressed. Circuit locating involves touching a reflex point and testing an IM. A change in IM response indicates involvement of the reflex point in the imbalance.

1. Use a clear circuit indicator muscle and circuit locate each of the following on both tester and testee. This is done by holding the points below with one hand and testing the IM.
- Ends of the collar bones near the sternal notch
- Tail bone
- Top and bottom lips

2. If any of these indicate, both partners must switch on.
3. Use the switching on exercises on page 21.

Relative Hydration

Water

An area often neglected is drinking water. Second only to air, water is a primary physical need. Our bodies are made up of about 70% water. We are dependent on the fluid flow of the different systems in our bodies. Every living cell requires water, just as it does nutrients and oxygen. Water acts as a solvent in the body, and the purer it is, free from minerals, softeners, and pollutants, the more body toxins can be let into it and the more nutrients it can carry to the body cells. There are no enzymes in rocks. Our mineral consumption should come from the living foods we eat -vegetables, fruits, grains, and meats. Animal trainers know to give their animals the purest possible water. Human beings deserve the same kind of treatment.

A healthy person should drink a minimum of 1/3 of an ounce of water for every pound of body weight, and at least double that in times of stress or illness. This means drinking at least 6- 8 glasses of water each day. A healthy person can easily handle up to five gallons of water a day. This means pure, distilled water. Coffee, tea, fruit juice, milk and other liquids don't count. They are processed in the body as food, whereas what the body needs is water. We can't substitute other liquids for water any more than we would want to fill the battery in the car with milk, the steam iron with tomato juice, or wash the walls with coffee.

For good performance, clarity of thinking, proper mind/body function, and smooth movement of the muscles, the body depends greatly on water. Without pure water the body's electrical system is impaired and the lymph system and organ function suffers. We say that a person is Relatively dehydrated on a subtle energy level if indicated by the test. This means that there is an energetic issue related to water. This may or may not relate to our physical level of hydration. When we drink water, we may not immediately be re-hydrated, but now the information is in the system that water is available. Now our natural thirst may be activated, or we may be more aware of it, or distinguish thirst from hunger or other cravings (Try drinking water first if you have excessive hunger or cravings! Water is often what your body is really crying out for!)

Ask the person to tug a tuft of their hair and test the IM
Locked = no relative/energetic dehydration indicated
Unlocked = hydration may be needed

Balancing technique for dehydration:
Both people have a drink of water. Then retest.

Pretests- Hydration

Touch for Health Muscle Testing or Monitoring

Even after 30 years of developing and teaching TFH, there remains some mystery about the phenomenon of muscle testing. TFH muscle testing is a mechanical skill which can be learned by anyone, but what the test means, and what we do about it, has more to do with the context of the muscle testing relationship, between two people, than it does with the precise observation of individual muscle response. The muscle test gives us an immediate, subjective (though objectively observable) and personally meaningful measurement that allows us access to powerful techniques to effect change and reinforce that change physically, mentally, emotionally, and spiritually in the whole Soul. For the most part, we are not measuring the gross physical strength of the muscle, but rather, *monitoring* the muscle response as an indication of changes in our energy. TFH muscle testing is both a bio-feedback mechanism which gives us subtle indications of how our life energy is effected on multiple levels, and it is also a concrete exercise which taps into the neuromuscular system to balance the physical posture. What each person experiences and learns through muscle testing depends on the beliefs that they both have *individually and collectively*. These beliefs are usually *implicit* and not explicitly discussed.

The Touch for Health System of muscle testing and energy balancing is used to achieve the following goals:

1. **Gain insight** into and AWARENESS of subtle changes in the Whole Person, the Whole Soul. This awareness involves:
    • An initial sense of one's overall sense of Wellness, balance, energy facilitation/inhibition
    • A subtle proprioceptive sense of muscle function and response (awareness of the physical sensation of a muscle's position and action)
    • Subtle CHANGES in proprioceptive sense of muscle function and response

• Corresponding changes in posture, attitude, emotion, mental functioning, etc.

2. The purpose of developing this awareness is to allow the person being balanced to feel **greater wholeness** on all levels of the Soul and have an improved integration within the whole person as well as socially, environmentally and in context of their lived life.

3. Restore postural balance, balance gait impairment, improve range of motion, & improve strength and energy

4. Achieve homeostasis of the various systems to allow the healing system to do its job more effectively

5. Assist the person seeking help to recognize imbalances, which may allow changes in function, feeling, and behavior that facilitate the prevention or delay of the frank onset of pathological processes

6. Assist one another to be aware of the Touch for Health model of healing, and the implicit assumptions of other healing models in order to have clear goals and expectations and achieve a maximum benefit when we seek help from any other person, particularly a health professional

7. Assist one another to be aware of the belief systems of our personal/cultural life and to see where they may be in conflict with our purposes and goals.

The phenomenon of inhibition or facilitation of muscles, before and after TFH intervention, is directly observable and relatively easy to experience for the tester and the person being tested. With a little bit of experience and practice, anyone can see changes in muscle response, and more importantly, in the overall being of the person whose muscles are tested and whose energy is balanced, particularly in the individual's own "before and after" sense of Wellness.

TFH Muscle Testing

Using this system allows you to evaluate the flow of energy in the meridians. Testing the relative strength of a particular muscle that is related to a particular meridian gives us an indication of meridian energy. Whether the muscle locks within a specific range of motion indicates the flow of energy to the muscle through its related meridian. By balancing the energy flow through use of various touch reflexes you can facilitate the natural healing process and enhance the natural biological recovery. And by confirming the shift in our energy by re-testing the muscle, we can reinforce the positive changes with a concrete, physical experience of the facilitated muscle response.

First, we need to learn the mechanical task of how to test a muscle. It takes some practice to develop the sensory-motor skills to feel the slight difference between a muscle that locks into position, and an inhibited muscle which does not "lock" or may feel "mushy", "shaky", "weak" or just not functioning at all within the range of the test. Arms, legs, or even the whole torso is positioned so that individual muscles are relatively isolated in a position of maximum contraction. The muscle is then gently moved through its full range of motion to enhance the person's sense of the muscle function and to "cue up" the meridian related to the muscle/function being tested.

After positioning the limb/muscle so that the muscle is the prime mover, we take it through its range of motion. Then, starting with the muscle in its most contracted position, we pull or push against the limb with about two pounds of pressure, for about two seconds, to see if the muscle "locks" in position, *within a range of about two inches*. This differs from other muscle testing systems in which the focus is on the gross physical strength of a muscle through its entire range of motion. In TFH, we are not really testing the strength of the muscle, but rather *monitoring* the response of the muscle in different contexts.

Whenever you agree to help another person using TFH and muscle testing, there are a number of things you need to consider to be the most effective helper.

TFH Muscle Testing

- Consider yourself the junior partner in the relationship—Your job is to assist the other person become more aware of themselves.

- Always tell the person that is being tested that they can stop the process at any time by saying the word stop or another agreed upon signal. If you are directing someone to touch you, be sure that they agree to stop when you say.

- Before doing any physical touching, check if there is any physical or medical condition that prohibits certain kinds of touching or movements. If someone is injured, you'll want to know ahead of time so that you don't exacerbate the problem. You may be able to work around an injury, or simply work gently with sore muscles, but you may need to do only light touch or simply refrain from trying to help the person in any physical way.

- Be sure you have mutual consent to what you will be doing. Explain the reflex point and its location in as clear and specific terms as possible, and don't hesitate to say stop if you're uncomfortable.

- Position yourself and the person being tested in ways that are safe and comfortable for you both. Do not use awkward postures that feel strained and risk injury to either yourself or the person you are testing.

- The person/muscle being tested must be stabilized to get an accurate test. For example, when pulling on an arm, it may be necessary to hold the opposite shoulder to counteract the tendency to turn the body. This will often eliminate confusion in test results and protect from unnecessary strain as the person attempts to maintain their posture while focusing on a subtle test.

- Apply an even, gradually increasing pressure, not a sudden "surprise" to the person/muscle. By starting with an almost imperceptible pressure and gradually increasing, you may find that you can sense muscle inhibition/facilitation with a very light touch. However, be sure to use enough pressure so that both participants can feel the muscle response. In the TFH model, the person being balanced is the authority, so even if the "tester" senses a muscle

TFH Muscle Testing

response, the test is not considered "valid" until both participants agree.

- It is not necessary to apply more than two pounds of pressure, as the test is used to indicate subtle differences in muscle response—not to see if one person can overpower the other.

- Testing for more than two seconds can often fatigue a muscle in isolation and cause it to give way.

- If the muscle response seems wobbly or mushy, or the muscle does not seem to lock into place within about two inches, this indicates that energy probably is not balanced within the related meridian. Go ahead and consider this an indication that an improvement can be made. Look for small improvements in muscle "locking" in the maximum contraction position. (The improvements may be dramatic!)

- Stop testing if the person has pain when you are testing them. Consider any pain, whether in the tested muscle or in some other place, an indication of inhibited energy flow and move on to the correction. pain in another muscle may indicate the muscle being tested is "recruiting" other muscles. Since the muscle test is designed to put synergistic muscles at a disadvantage, it's easier to injure a related muscle if you ignore pain.

- Stop testing if YOU have a pain when doing the test. Each individual needs to be aware and responsible for him or herself. You cannot be as effective if you do not listen to yourself and protect yourself. If you have a pain doing the test, your posture will show it and may have an effect on the outcome. You also risk injury and your ability to be of further help to anyone.

- If the person being tested feels an improvement, the person assisting in the testing must not deny that improvement. Re-testing following intervention gives more accuracy to the test when doubt is present.

TFH Muscle Testing

Muscle Testing FAQ's
Short Answers to Frequently Asked Questions
Q. What should the person being tested feel?
A. Both people participating in the test are looking for subtle changes in the flow of energy. The person being tested is the authority in determining this. The person being tested should try to be aware of their sense of comfort and ability to place their limb in the test position; whether there is any pain associated with the position or the effort to maintain the position during the test; and whether the muscle seems to be "locking" into position easily, or with great effort.

- It is very beneficial to try to have a proprioceptive sense of the location of the actual muscle and feel its contraction in the test position.

- The context of the muscle test is an awareness and facilitation of the sense of self, Wellness and facilitation and flow of energy in the whole Soul. The purpose of muscle testing and energy balancing is to facilitate and reinforce this process, and so it is very beneficial for the person being tested to have some awareness of how they are feeling as a whole even as they are focussing on subtle and refined aspects of muscles.

Q. What is happening when we test the muscle in a particular position?
A. 1. We are refining proprioception of the muscle for the person (the ability to know the position of the muscle without seeing it, only feeling the muscle and its action), both in terms of the physical location of the muscle and the function of the muscle through a range of motion.
2. We are isolating the muscle, to some extent, from other muscles.
3. We are refining our indicator from general to specific, from, "How do you feel as a whole?" to, "How does the energy seem to be flowing within this narrow range?"
4. We are preparing to assess balance in various aspects of the whole Soul by inference as they are associated with the specific muscle.

Q. If we are not testing JUST the muscle, and our interest is really much more focused on subtle energy changes, why do we bother to be so precise in our testing?

A. The physical paradigm is incomplete, but it is very powerful to get as full and exact a sense of muscle location, position, contraction and facilitation as possible. By finely tuning our muscle testing, we promote an attitude of finely tuning our awareness of all of the aspects of the whole Soul. However, even an imprecise muscle test can be very effective for biofeedback and noticing subtle change.

Q. I was talking to a (medical doctor, chiropractor, physical therapist, kinesiologist…) and I was told that the TFH test is not the correct test for the muscle that is named. Shouldn't we alter the tests in the book so that they will be medically/scientifically correct?

A. No. Although we have done some refining of the TFH muscle tests over the years, and kinesiologists will always be devising new and varied muscle tests, the 42 tests in the TFH system have been very useful and effective for thousands of people over the course of 30 years and will continue to be so. In TFH we are more concerned with the ability to observe change in the muscle, and subsequent changes in the whole person. The muscle tests, as they are described in the TFH manual, this pocketbook, TFH reference materials and classes, have a very high correlation with the reflexes/energy-meridians in the TFH system. Whatever we choose to name the muscle tests, they are the correct tests for our purposes.

We are less concerned with exact correlation with anatomy texts, or kinesiology manuals. There is variation from manual to manual, text to text, school to school, and most importantly, from person to person. It is most accurate to find the position of maximum contraction, where the person can become aware of the functioning of the muscle, for the unique individual we are helping.

Q. Isn't the body the final authority for what we need? Isn't the result of the Muscle test the most important information?
A. No. The individual person seeking energy balancing is the authority in the Touch For Health system. Whether the person assisting in testing has a different opinion, or the muscle test seems to contradict a person's beliefs about themselves, it is up to the Individual to contemplate the true meaning of his or her own responses and changes in muscular, postural, emotional, mental or spiritual function. TFH is only used to assist and facilitate this personal process.

The test is one piece of information, and one exchange in a relationship and process of assessment at a moment in the life of a person. As the poet said, "It is like a finger pointing towards the moon. Do not concentrate on the finger or you will miss all that heavenly glory." The result of a muscle test is only an indication. It points toward meaning in an individual person's life. Don't get so carried away by the muscle that you forget it's NOT SEPARATE from the person, their energy, their thoughts, emotions, intentions, dreams, beliefs, etc.

This contrasts with a diagnostic model where an expert takes biomedical measurements or tests for disease agents, and then tells you how you are doing. In the Touch for Health system, the individual subjective sense of well-being is the primary measurement.

Q. How can I test myself?
A. When you don't have anyone nearby you can ask to help you, you can benefit simply by noticing how you feel before and after working the reflexes, as with Zip-ups or Switching-on. But ideally, you will get the "touch" part of TFH by asking someone to help you by pushing on your arms and legs. They don't need to already "know" TFH for you to show them the range of motion and direction of the muscle test, and you can direct them on how much pressure you prefer. This is generally very effective.

Muscle Testing FAQ's

Muscle Testing & Balancing Tips

Cautionary Note:
If any technique seems like it "doesn't work", DO NOT be hasty to give up and try a different reflex or technique. There is probably a reason why you have not found the expected response. Usually, if both people make an effort to be more aware of the details of the technique, and look for slight changes or improvements, the techniques will work. When working with balancing the subtle energy, small changes may be all that will be necessary for big improvement in the whole person, the Soul.

On the Other Hand:
There is no danger if you want to stop in the middle of a balancing. If time or comfort requires you to skip, postpone or discontinue a particular technique or balancing, you will still get the benefit of the techniques you do complete.

After we work with a reflex, we expect some difference in the muscle we are testing. When we retest, the muscle will be
1. The Same, 2. worse or 3. better.

1. The Same: If the muscle doesn't seem to improve after working a particular reflex,
A. Encourage the person to be more present in the process. Ask them to involve their awareness in the location and the feeling of the particular muscle.
B. Double check the test position, range of motion and amount of pressure used.
C. See what **metaphors** are related to the muscle/meridian/element and think about how these might relate to your life/goal.
D. Try to be aware of subtle differences. If you notice even a slight improvement, consider this an indication, even if it's not "completely locking". If there's even slight improvement then go to **3. Better.**

E. If you don't seem to be getting any change, you can also try **jiggling** the muscle to "wake it up".

F. Finally, review your pretests for **Accurate Indicator Muscles** and the other pretests. Taking the time to do these pretests will help a lot. Review step 4 of the AIM test for things you can do when you are not getting the expected muscle response.

2. Worse: If the muscle seems to get even weaker after each balancing reflex,

A. Check for over energy in the meridian by holding one hand on the alarm point for the muscle/meridian, and testing an Indicator Muscle.

B. If a strong muscle goes weak while holding the alarm point, go to the related acupressure holding points for Sedation to draw the excess energy into another meridian.

C. Retest the muscle and it will probably be strong now.

3. Better: If even slight improvement is noticed, then **challenge** by placing one hand over the reflex point and re-testing the muscle.

A. *If the muscle improves* while holding the reflex, that is, the muscle gets stronger, then work this same reflex some more.

B . *If the muscle gets weaker* while holding the reflex, then go on to the next strengthening technique for the muscle.

C. *If the muscle is just the same* while holding the reflex, then move on to the next muscle test.

Each session is an attempt to facilitate the balance of the subtle energy. This is a continuous and ongoing process within each Soul. All of the various factors of our lives are always inter-relating in a dynamic and cyclical balance of the subtle energies. The Touch for Health balancing process assists in releasing blocks in the natural, intelligent design of the healing system, to improve the continuous flow of energy. This allows each Soul to fulfill their missions, using all their talents to ultimately reach their destiny. Balancing and rebalancing is an ongoing process. It is Ok to use as much of the TFH energy balancing procedure you will give yourself time for.

Testing & Balancing Tips

About Challenging

After balancing, we want to be sure that we have done enough to keep the muscle locked. After you have re-tested a previously weak/unlocked muscle and it seems strong have the person place their hand on the points you just worked on and re-test the muscle. If the muscle goes weak when you do this, go on to the next strengthening technique for that muscle and repeat the re-test/challenge process for that technique. If the muscle stays strong on the challenge, you are finished strengthening that muscle. Go on to your next muscle test.

Challenging Procedure:

1. In the case of bilateral weakness, use the related spinal reflexes.
2. Retest both sides. If both lock, move on to the next muscle test. If only one locks, correct with the neurolymphatic reflex (NL).
3. Retest the muscle. If it now locks …
4. Challenge by touching the NL while testing the muscle. If the muscle locks, move on to the next muscle test. If the muscle unlocks while holding the NL point…
5. Use the corresponding neurovascular holding (NV) points, and retest while holding the NL.
6. If strong, challenge the NV points by re-testing while holding a NV point. If it is strong on the challenge, go on to the next muscle test. If it does not stay locked, move to the next reflex.
7. Continue working through the balancing techniques until the muscle test stays locked after challenging all reflexes.

Basic Order of Reflexes:
Spinal Reflex,
Neurolymphatic Reflex,
Neurovascular Reflex,
Meridian Tracing,
Origin and Insertion Techniques,
Acupressure Holding Points

Tips: About Challenging

The order of the strengthening techniques, as with most all of the TFH system, was developed on the basis of ease, simplicity, and efficiency. This is the order that was found, through thousands of balancings, to produce the best results in the shortest amount of time. As you become adept at the techniques, and adapt your own style and favorite routines, you may find that it is easier or more effective for you to do the techniques in a different order, or use **Circuit Location** to determine which reflex to start with.

Circuit Locating
In TFH we use reflex systems which may be associated with particular physiological systems - spinal reflexes, neurolymphatics, neurovasculars, meridians, etc- but we focus on the way these reflexes can positively affect a muscle response as an indication of the flow of energy.

Energetically speaking, when a muscle locks, we know that we have an "intact" circuit. Physiologically, this means that sensory nerves have recorded our testing pressure and sent this information back to the spinal cord and brain. This has responded by sending information down the motor nerve to tell the muscles to lock. If the muscle does not lock, we know that somewhere in the energy circuitry an imbalance is occurring.

When using the "14 muscle balance, fix as you go" model, we use the corrections, in a set order until the muscles lock and stay locked when challenging the reflex. We can also circuit locate before we work the reflexes to see which reflexes will facilitate the muscle. It may be that tracing the meridian will be most effective at the moment, so if we start there we can save time compared to working SR, NL, NV, and then the meridian.

E.S.R.- Emotional Stress Release

A very effective balancing technique in TFH is Emotional Stress Release - E.S.R. This simple method allows one to feel they are coping in times of stress, trauma, overload, accident, pressure from work or relationships etc. The technique requires a light touch on the frontal eminences, the bumps on the forehead between the hairline and the eyebrows, above the eyes. (These are the neurovascular points for the Stomach Meridian, see the Stomach Meridian Reference Page) The light touch on this reflex point has a harmonizing effect on the energy of the forebrain where new options and ideas are processed. It is here that the brain can be creative and think of new solutions without being overwhelmed by emotion.

In times of stress, our usual response is "fight or flight", the way we have learned to survive. Translated today, that often means anger or fear, and a reaction based on past experiences. Using E.S.R., we can think of new solutions and choose to change the way we react to stress.

How to use E.S.R.

Do the usual pre-checks, and ideally do at least a 14 muscle balance. Use a strong indicator muscle. (The pectoralis major clavicular is particularly good, since it relates to the Stomach meridian. When we are emotionally traumatized, the Stomach meridian is directly affected, hence we feel churned up and sometimes nauseous.) Test while the person thinks of their problem. If the muscle unlocks, suggest that the person hold their frontal eminences (or you can do it for them) while thinking about their stress. These are usually slight bulges on the forehead, directly over the eyes, half way between the eyebrows and the natural hairline. It may be necessary to think through this several times. When the person feels they have held long enough, retest the indicator muscle while thinking of the stress. It will lock when the process is complete. We have not changed the memory of the trauma or stress, we have changed the reaction to the memory of the trauma or stress. This can also allow us to react differently to similar experiences in the future.

Since the E.S.R. points are neurovascular points, and effect subtle changes in vascular circulation, particularly in the brain, it is helpful to engage diverse areas of the brain- and make the visualization more vivid- by asking the person to contemplate aspects of their goals or stressful issues through the 5 senses. You might ask, "If your goal had a smell, what would it be? What color do you see when you think about the stressful issue? When you see yourself achieving your goal, what sounds, voices, words do you hear? What physical, bodily, tactile sensation do you have? As you develop your sensitivity, you will be able to feel a pulse in each of the points. For each aspect of the stressful memory/situation, holding the points will bring the pulses back into sync. As you contemplate different aspects, the pulses may go out of sync and come back into sync.

E.S.R. can work in times of simple mental block e.g. exams, interviews, overwhelm, confrontations, and for accidents or trauma etc. It is also helpful for relieving stress related to past experiences, or anticipated future events.

Safe Place
When using E.S.R. to defuse traumatic experiences, it may be necessary to set up a "safe place". This may be real or imagined, and allows the person to take "time out" from the process if necessary. An IM should lock when the person thinks about their safe place. (If using a "safe place", ask the person to indicate when they are ready to resume the process.) Sometimes if an emotion comes up and it is overwhelming, we can ask the person to think of something neutral, like "fresh bread". They can then choose to work with the emotion, or set it aside for another time or a different setting. Some people are comfortable working through tears, but we respect a person's right to stop or not to go there.

Emotional Stress Release

Goal Setting/ Goal Balancing

The TFH balance is more than just a structural assessment of the body's musculature to see if the left and right sides of the body are working equally or if the front and back muscles are working in harmony. The status of the muscles also gives us a sense of the balance in the meridian system and can give us insight into the overall functioning of the person in their current context.

We have found that for each different goal that we have, there is a different pattern of energy as indicated by the muscle tests. And we have also found that if we balance the energy related to a particular goal, the subsequent shifts in posture, attitude, energy etc. can be a profound and dramatic help in reaching that goal. Your goal can be as simple and general as improving your energy balance and enhancing your sense of Wellness. Your goal can be related to pain, symptoms, etc. but it is more powerful if it is framed in terms of a positive outcome that you whole-heartedly want, rather than simply in terms of what you do not want. It can be improved range of motion, improved physical performance, personal best in an exam, a job interview, or any activity that may be stressful, including something in the past that still affects us. We can balance our energy to achieve our peak performance and personal best in any area of our life.

Basic Goal Balancing Protocol
1. Do any pre-checks you normally do.

2. You may want to do a preliminary balance, "in the clear" with no goal in mind other than starting with a clear baseline. This way, you can see a pattern that is more exclusively related to your goal. Once you are confident in accepting the "muscle picture" goals produce, there is no need to do a preliminary balance. You can make every balance a goal balance and really put power into your TFH.

3. Frame your goal as a positive statement as a fact in present time. For example: " I am good at muscle testing and balancing", or "I learn new skills easily and readily apply them in daily life."

4. As you state your goal, simultaneously test an indicator muscle, such as the anterior deltoid. The muscle will probably not lock, indicating that there is some energy blockage that we can work with to facilitate the achievement of your goal. If the indicator muscles do not unlock, make sure you are "present" and thinking of your goal and the muscle test. You may need to rephrase your goal or think of a particular aspect to find an indicator muscle change. Or simply recognize and reinforce the fact that you are already in balance for that particular goal!

5. Now all of the subsequent muscle testing and balancing relates to the goal in mind. It can be helpful to continue to think about the goal through the balancing, but the energy pattern and balancing will generally relate to the goal that was stated before the balance. This pattern will usually be quite different than the pattern that we found, "in the clear".

6. After balancing all of the muscles/meridians, restate your goal and retest your indicator muscle. The IM should now lock, indicating that we have balanced our energy related to the goal.
* If there is still stress on the goal statement, use E.S.R. (light holding on the forehead) to clear any residual stress. Now your IM should lock, and you will generally feel a sense of relief and an improved attitude and energy towards your goal.

Further Balancing
You can test and balance for several goals one after another. Not feeling good about yourself? Balance for a statement like, " I accept myself as a beautiful, loving and lovable person." Now wait for the positive results. It is amazing how quickly they follow.

Goal Balancing with Five Element Emotion Metaphors

There is frequently a great deal of emotion involved with our life goals, and it is important that the emotional component is also taken into consideration during the balance. One easy way to begin to incorporate the 5 Element Metaphors into our balancing is to muscle test to find which emotion is related to your goal. This also makes the goal balance more powerful by emphasizing the emotional aspect of the balancing.

1. Do any pre-checks and set a goal, as in the basic goal balancing.

2. Find the Emotion.
a. First, look at the metaphor "pie" found on the Five Elements Reference page. Look at the "slice" of pie related to emotions. This will give you the emotions related to each of the five elements (Fear for Water, Grief for Metal, Sympathy/Empathy for Earth, Joy for Fire, and Anger for Wood)

b. Muscle test while saying each of the emotions aloud. A switched off IM will identify the element where the stressful emotion is located. You can further muscle test to find out if the emotion is related to self, others, things or circumstances. Often, it's easy to see how the identified emotion is tied to the goal, but sometimes it is a mystery to contemplate.

3. Now do your energy balancing, either fix-as-you-go, or assessment.

4. Recheck the goal and the Emotion after the balance. Clear any further imbalance with E.S.R..

Goal Balancing with Emotions

In Depth Goal Balancing with a Holistic Wellness Approach

Goal setting is a focussed, manageable way to:
- Assess and develop and be mindful of our sense of a purpose,
- Remember or discern our talents, gifts and skills,
- Discover what we are passionate about and what fills us with energy,
- Increase our sense of balance and harmony with our purposes and desires,
- Balance, focus and direct the flow of energy towards our purposes,
- Measure and monitor our experience of wholeness and personal bests,
- Bring "online" a maximum of mental, physical, emotional and spiritual factors related to our goals, problems, issues or pains,
- Come into harmony with our environment, or find a new environment in which we will naturally thrive,
- Clear negative influences, and draw on the positive resources of our past, present and future

The Wellness approach to goal setting assumes that our fundamental challenge in life is fulfilling our full potential, and that the resources for fulfilling our potential are within us. Through dialogue, we can make available the information and the integrated flow of energy necessary for our natural unfolding as a unique being. This is an ongoing and dynamic process. It is a process of (re)discovering our core/central life values and purpose(s), which frees us to see and focus our energy on what REALLY matters. Goal setting is a mental process, which in and of itself helps to balance our energy and make our goals more real and attainable, but also creates an energy pattern that we can then balance to create profound shifts in energy, posture, attitude and function.

What we do to assist each other is to find mental incongruities or stress and energetic blocks or imbalances. We then increase our awareness, clear stress and blocks, and enhance and balance the flow of energy. Part of our hypothesis is that this process of enhancing energy flow involves making information available to the innate intelligence enabling the natural process of healing, growth and adaptation needed to fulfill our purposes. The crucial factor in making all of the incredible parallel systems work together seems to be our conscious awareness and VISION. When we talk about all of the different aspects of our vision, we increase brain activity and the "multi-tasking"- parallel processing of the brain (from which we infer a similar level of activity in the overall physical, conscious, emotional, and spiritual intelligence systems of the Soul).

We all have special, unique gifts and talents. When we can know and utilize our personal skills there is a sense of fulfillment that makes our tasks and our work a reward in itself. Getting our energy balanced regularly can help us recognize the path that is nourishing to us, and see the things that are blocking our health. Goal balancing is one way of feeling that pull to what is uniquely right for each of us. Even when facing a "failure" we can reframe our experience as guidance toward our life purpose, or telos. As an organism in an ecosystem, you will thrive in some roles and relationships more than others. But we can also overcome obstacles and adapt to adversity if we see a purpose that is truly important to us and harness our passion and energies to persevere.

The goal-setting and balancing process helps us to explore the future that we anticipate or expect, consciously or unconsciously. When we can break out of the straitjacket of our own assumptions we can think creatively and positively, even in the face of seemingly dire circumstances. Use of 5 Element and other metaphors liberates us from habitual, linear thinking and helps us to see aspects of ourselves that we may be "blind" to. We allow the possibility that our present problems can also be opportunities and that our present obstacles and limitations can be transcended. We ask not only what is, but also what could be and most of all expand our opportunities and abilities to make conscious choices.

Many of us feel that our future is shaped by our past, but we need to recognize that our images of the future also help shape our beliefs about the past. When we have a different image of the future this will invite a different image of the past. In order to do this we must compare our beliefs about the past, our beliefs about the present, and our expectations and hopes for the future. When these beliefs are in conflict, or converge on a negative image, we find subtle energy imbalances as shown by muscle testing. Balancing these muscles and contemplating the associated metaphors can facilitate change in our thinking, in our feeling, and in our actions.

We can choose which elements of our past will help to shape our future. We can recall those moments when we have been in touch with our own Wellness, our wholeness and our holiness, using our memory and imagination as a reference for equilibrium in our subtle energies. As we balance our energy towards these positive images we find it easier to utilize our talents, and fulfill our destinies in a manner of our own choosing.

The biofeedback mechanism of muscle testing is a powerful reinforcement of positive change. Thinking in metaphorical terms about our goals and our difficulties breaks us out of rigid conceptions of our circumstances and possibilities. As we become more sensitive to subtle changes in our muscles, our postures, our attitudes and mental states, and develop creative and intuitive insights into our life, we improve our ability to adapt to our environments, overcome adversity and meet our most valued and desired goals.

In-Depth Goal Balancing

Remembering Wellness Goal-setting Protocol

When we remember Wellness, our aim is to assist ourselves, our family, friends, and clients to BE WHO WE ARE, WHO WE WERE MEANT, CREATED, SPOKEN FORTH TO BE. We use discussion, listening, questioning and TFH energy balancing techniques to be supportive in a process of becoming aware of, developing, and coming into balance with our own unique purpose(s) in life.

1. Establish Setting/Understanding

• Each Soul is in charge of his or her own goal(s). The individual Soul is the authority in his or her own Wellness process.

• *Establish a cooperative encounter/process* in which each individual decides for themselves and says start or stop, more or less, yes or no, harder or softer, now, later, or never.

LISTEN: Acknowledge the person first. Allow all participants to be themselves and express their own purpose(s), pain and meaning. Is this YOUR purpose, or one which someone else, or circumstances have imposed on you?

• *Use Active Listening* to clarify what the person feels, what they believe about their thoughts, pains, emotions, and other aspects of their experience of life. What do they believe is the cause of their feelings? What meaning does this have for them?

2. Set a Goal, Listen to the call

• *What do you want* (better) in your life? What performance, activity, or (emotional, practical, physical) problem or issue do you want to address in the goal-setting, energy-balancing process?

• *Is it appropriate for YOU?* Is it a goal you can own, accept for yourself, feel like you deserve. (Not forced, no shoulds). Is it at an appropriate *comfort level* (NOT so small as to be insignificant, and not a goal that is really just going to stress you out, or is completely Utopian) Is it in keeping with your values and beliefs?

- *Engage the WHOLE SOUL* towards a goal that you can be enthusiastic about, that you **genuinely, (whole-heartedly) WANT.**

3. Take a History

- *Establish rapport* and acknowledge the person as a whole Soul within the context of their whole life and history, rather than a "patient", sick person, or "body" (some object you will work upon).
- This can be an in-depth, clinical history or just a getting acquainted gloss of biographical info. and background of goal/issue.

4. Extend the Goal

- When you reach your goal, *what will it mean* in your lived life? *How will your life be better?* What changes might it create? What are some possible outcomes, results, consequences, and alterquences?
- If the goal is to stop doing something, or to reduce pain, *see if the goal can be reframed in a positive light*. What will you be able to do or have in your life when you've resolved the problem. What will you do when with the time previously spent on the dropped behavior?

5. Remember Wellness

- Remember to be well. Remember how it feels to be well. Think of a time when you had that same feeling, that same experience that you want to have again. Use your imagination (EVEN IF YOU HAVE NO ACTUAL RECOLLECTION) to get as vivid a sense as possible of how it will be when you've reached your goal.
- Appreciate the meaning of pain, symptoms. The full experience of our range of motions and emotions is part of living a full, whole life.
- Have faith. Act "as if" you know that your goal is already accomplished. Now it simply needs to unfold.
- Set it up. Make note of your planned outcomes in measurable steps.

Goal Balancing Protocol

6. Make an Assessment

• Take a moment to notice how you feel. Stand up, get a sense of your balance (have your partner observe your posture, how you're moving, your ranges of motion). *Assess your range of motion in various postures.*

• How will you feel when you achieve your goal? Make a mental note, or jot down your observations. Make assessments between "0 and 10" on analog scales, measuring your subjective sense of where you are now as compared to worst/best case scenario. You can rate your level of pain, or your level of functioning at a given task, or just rate how you feel, or feel about something.

• Frame your goal as a positive statement as a fact in present time. For example: " I am good at muscle testing and balancing", or " I learn new skills easily and readily apply them in daily life."

• As you state your goal, simultaneously test an indicator muscle, such as the anterior deltoid. The muscle will probably not lock, indicating that there is some energy blockage that we can work with to facilitate the achievement of your goal. If the indicator muscles do not unlock, make sure you are "present" and thinking of your goal and the muscle test. You may need to rephrase your goal or think of a particular aspect to find an indicator muscle change. Or simply recognize and reinforce the fact that you are already in balance for that particular goal! *You can also find an attractor number-- see the comments following this outline, on page 59.*

7. Test the Supraspinatus

• Stress on the Supraspinatus indicates a "good goal". There is some stress related to your goal, and so it's something we can help clear through energy balancing.

• If the supraspinatus does not show an imbalance, try rephrasing the goal until you've brought the issue (and the related energy systems) "on line", or consider that you may already be in balance for this goal.

Goal Balancing Protocol

8. Do Something

• Ideally, do at least a 14-muscle balance. Checking at least one muscle for each of the major meridians will give you a holistic balancing of the energy system. You might also contemplate related Chinese 5-Element Metaphors, meditate, go for a walk, consult with your loved ones, go see a healer, therapist, doctor, etc. It is often very helpful to get your energy balanced before and/or after any therapy.

9. Notice Change - Re-Assess

• Take some time to **put your experience into words**.

• Verbalize the positive changes in how you are thinking and feeling (physically, emotionally, and spiritually).

• **Clarify** and quantify with a new assessment on an **analog scale**.

• Be sure that you **Re-test to affirm your energy balance** in the whole Soul.

• **Reinforce your experience** of positive change by listening to your partner's observations and confirm those observations that are true for you.

10. Reassess Your Goal

• What parts of your goal have been transformed through the goal setting and energy balancing process?

• **SET IT UP** Decide and make note of the next time/schedule for reassessing your goal, reassessing your Soul, and doing something to balance your energies.

WE RECOMMEND A ROUTINE OF QUICK DAILY BALANCINGS, ideally at the same time each day to keep in the habit. Then do in-depth goal-setting and balancing whenever an important issue or performance comes up, or whenever you're feeling "down", whether it's due to illness, depression, set-backs or just general listlessness and lethargy.

Goal Balancing Protocol

REMEMBERING WELLNESS Goal-Balancing Protocol
~ *Comments*

1. Establish setting/understanding
Who's in charge? Who's the authority? [remember: Only you know exactly how you feel and what you think and what you believe]

Goal setting can help clarify expectations of all of the participants in the therapeutic encounter. Your assumptions or the assumptions of the person you are helping may be inaccurate or conflicting. Do you know what is most important to your friend, student, client, patient? Perhaps the person you're working with assumes that you will automatically understand "what is wrong" and how best to "get it fixed", or they have their own pre-conceived idea of the best way to fix it, but assume that you are already in agreement with them, "It goes without saying".

Determining what you are being asked to do is an important first step. If you are acting as a holistic practitioner, what are your goals for your clients? If you are getting help for yourself from another person(professional or family member, acquaintance or friend) what do you want the outcome to be in your lived life? What will you be able to do that you are not now doing? What do you want to accomplish? It is often helpful to verbalize your goals in detail and talk them over, but there is also a great benefit in thinking about your goals internally, and simply having your energy balanced for what you're thinking about, without having to share it.

It can be a great relief to the person you're assisting to know that they can work towards a "small" goal, and needn't even verbally state their goal if they're not comfortable doing so, or simply wish to keep their goal to themselves. "Listening" to a person may involve respecting their desire to keep silent. On the other hand, the dialogue process of goal setting often opens up personal vistas for potential life change. When people get in touch with a goal for their lived life that they can

Goal Protocol ~ Comments

truly be enthusiastic about, it often creates a sense of joy and hope for fulfillment and change which charges their whole Soul with a transformative, creative, healing energy.

2. Set a Goal: IDENTIFY THE ISSUE
What do you want (better)?/ Listen to the call

A goal can be a momentary desire for a simple accomplishment or it can be a goal that will take all of your energies and life commitment. What performance, activity, problem, or SYMPTOM (emotional, practical, functional, physical, mental, spiritual) do you want to improve? Sometimes our physical pains and postures and our inhibitions and restrictions of movement can tell us something about what we do or don't want to be doing, so our life goals might flow out of simpler, immediate functional goals. Or we may have a long-term goal that is blocked or made more difficult by physical symptoms that we try to ignore. If we take a moment to listen to ourselves, the messages that our symptoms may represent, there is often a great insight into what we really want, as well as a relief from the pain.

If the goal is to stop doing something, or to reduce pain, see if the goal can be **reframed in a positive light.** Instead of simply "having less low-back pain" ask yourself, "what is it I WANT TO DO that the low back pain is preventing me from doing?" Maybe you want to be able to drive to your mother-in-law's home and give her a hug without back pain. That may raise multiple issues that may be involved in the low back pain. Is your relationship with your car seat working? (Do you have enough room? Do you feel ok about your car, or do you feel like you should have a new one?) How is your relationship with your mother-in-law?

Goal setting allows greater healing than digging out "what is wrong". It is a very effective addition to the healing process. We want people to really wonder and make choices about what they really want. We want them to wonder about the meaning of life and what would give their lives meaning. The process of making choices that are truthful for the Soul becomes clearer when we get the Soul moving through its natural cycles by balancing the meridian energy.

DON'T SHOULD ON YOURSELF: Set a goal that is appropriate for you, and **that you can own** (not forced, no shoulds). ESTABLISH AN APPROPRIATE LEVEL OF RISK, at an appropriate comfort level (NOT too easy or insignificant, and not a goal that is really just going to stress you out, or is completely Utopian).

YOU CAN STOP ANY TIME if your level of comfort changes or you feel rising tears. You may stop any time and do the balance with or without a goal. Also, if at any point in a balancing the feelings or discussion is too unpleasant, you can stop and hold the frontal eminences as in the Emotional Stress Release technique. Depending on the comfort level of both people, you may either work through the tears, if that feels right for you, or think of "fresh bread", stop thinking about what's distressing you at the moment and get clear.

More important than dwelling on what you don't want is thinking of a goal that you can be enthusiastic about, that you genuinely, **whole-heartedly WANT.** ENGAGE THE WHOLE SOUL TOWARDS A POSITIVE GOAL. Ultimately, the **desired outcome is more important than the complaint**. What feeling do you want to have when you are relieved of suffering? What specific activities will you be better able to perform? What will truly bring you joy and a sense of being fully alive?

Be careful of Utopianism: Recognize that, although you MAY have an instantaneous transformation/healing, it is often the natural process for things to change gradually. Your goal-setting helps to focus the DIRECTION of change, but you may not be able to fully address a given issue, or include all of the issues that are of concern to you in a single goal-setting/ energy balancing session. It's okay to approach a small part, take a small step. Addressing one aspect will have a positive influence on the whole.

You may need to ask yourself if your goal is to change someone else or to change yourself. Often, simply recognizing that you are trying to change someone else can lead to a lot of relief as you focus on what you do have power to change, which is your own attitude, posture and behavior.

You may feel conflicted about a goal. Part of you may really want the goal, but part of you may not want what goes with it. Getting balanced for your goal may help you to accept the sacrifices involved, or it may help you realize that it's not something you really want.

Where the goal is "fuzzy" or the enthusiasm for a positive goal is mushy, there may be some disassociation of the Soul with the actual life of the person. You may know in your head what your goal is supposed to be, but you aren't really living it, you aren't enlivened by your "own" purposes, perhaps because you don't really own them. If this is the case, it may be helpful to go back to your history and find out why you started on your particular path, or try to think of the first time you were aware that your goals were not energizing you.

Fishing for Issues
If I am assisting someone to set their goals and they seem to have no idea what they feel their goal should be I might use muscle testing to find a general area that is appropriate. I'll have the person say various words related to general categories such as family, money, sex, job, home, or work. When there is an inhibition of the muscle after saying the word, think about what comes to mind related to the word. The issue may not be the logical meaning of the word itself, but what you personally associate with it. Now that you have an issue in mind, formulate your goal related to the issue.

3. Take a History: Take a moment for "Getting to know you", establish rapport. Acknowledge the person as a whole Soul within the context of their whole life and history. Give them the role of "Thou", central authority in their own life, rather than "patient", sick person, or "body" (some object that you will work upon).

If this is the first time you've worked together, or if this is the first time you've worked on a particular issue, performance, problem, symptom, etc., it can be helpful to get some sense of the history. This can be an in depth, clinical case history, or just a brief gloss of a person's basic biographical information, or the basic background of the goal in question. Often, thinking back to the beginning of a career, or health issue, or a quest (and thinking about what else was happening in your life at the time) can give you clues to what you truly want, and help reintegrate your purposes with your current life.

4. Extend the Goal

Follow the goal to what it will mean in your lived life. When you achieve your goal, what will it do for you? What changes might it create, what outcomes, consequences, alterquences may result. Taking a moment to acknowledge possible or expected negative consequences, and then thinking of alternative outcomes can often relieve a lot of the stress associated with unacknowledged fear. And part of this fear may be related to positive outcomes, and the responsibilities that come with success. Envisioning all of the aspects of a desired outcome, and then balancing your energy can really transform how you feel about your tasks and how you function.

If your goal has to do with alleviating certain symptoms, you may want to look at the meaning of these symptoms in your life. What purpose are they serving? Are you required to have these symptoms to continue to receive certain benefits or compensation? Is there a more satisfying way to receive similar or greater benefits? Sometimes symptoms occur and we want to get rid of them without wondering what message may be found in the symptoms. When the symptoms are gone, what difference will it make in your life? What are the symptoms keeping you from doing that you want to do (or don't want to do)? We sometimes uncover motivations and goals that are unsaid, and perhaps unconscious. Sometimes we can logically, mentally see what we want, or what we don't want, but we seem locked in a pattern that is not fulfilling. Getting balanced for a goal that is true to your heart can often lead to dramatic shifts and new paths.

5. REMEMBER WELLNESS

Think of a time when you had that same feeling, same experience that you want to have again. If you can't remember a time when you had that, use your imagination to get as vivid a sense as possible of how it will be.

Remember to feel Well. Dedicate some of your energy to actually experiencing your feelings and being present in your experiences. Remember to make the choices that you feel good about, or that will nourish your Wellness (rather than simply ignoring your feelings and powering through).

Remember *how it felt* to feel Well. When was the last time you really felt well? When was the time you felt the most alive and in harmony? If you can't think of such a time, use your imagination to see what it might have been, or what it might be.

Remember How to feel Well. If you have an experience to draw on, you can often apply the same formula to reproduce the same feeling. Or you may need to a apply a completely new strategy to create your new Wellness, but balancing your energy with this reference may help **you remember or discover the steps you want to take. Imagine, HOW WILL IT FEEL?** Imagination is a clinical instrument to mobilize all of your interior resources towards a positive vision.

Appreciate the Meaning of Pain, Symptoms

The full experience of our range of motions and emotions is part of living a full, whole life. Sometimes if we stop trying to ignore pain and look at its meaning, particularly in the context of balancing our energy, there is a lot of relief. If you had a positive experience that also had some negative aspects or consequences, acknowledge whether having the same kind of positive experience is likely to also produce the negative part too.

Have Faith
"Go confidently in the direction of your dream. Act as if it is impossible to Fail."
---Thoreau
"As a man thinketh, in his heart, so IS he." ---Proverbs

Once you have the feeling that you can actually achieve your goal, you're much more likely to make it happen (and know it when you see it!) Act "as if" you know that your goal is already accomplished. Now it simply needs to unfold.
In Christianity, this is the principle of praying with the knowledge that your prayers will be answered. This is also seen in the power of positive affirmation statements in personal growth and change .

SET IT UP: Make note of your planned outcomes. How will you know that your goal is achieved? Break the goal into measurable steps. When will you be sure to check in on your goal to see that you're taking the steps. How will you celebrate each step and your final accomplishment?

6. Make an Assessment:
You may want to stand up, get a sense of your balance/posture, assess your range of motion in various postures. Add to this your own general sense of mood, posture, attitude, enthusiasm, etc It is very helpful to measure your overall sense of wellness, your enthusiasm, or any symptoms on an **analog scale**. This can be a simple horizontal line with zero at one end and 10 at the other. You will rate your goal(s)/symptom(s) somewhere along this continuum. You can get

creative with vertical scales, bar graphs, or circles that are divided by percentages. The most valuable assessments measure both subjective and objective aspects of your functioning and feeling.

Using analog scales has been recognized as an important method of understanding the pain phenomena. They are useful in noting the differences in pain in different circumstances,and in measuring and being AWARE of improvements (and having hope). Starting with a horizontal line, we can mark one end, "No Pain" and have the other end represent, "Worst Pain Ever". We mark the current pain on the scale both before and after balancing. Measuring the pain makes it more real, and possibly more excruciating as we become completely aware of it, but that same awareness seems to contribute greatly to the relief we feel.

In the same way, when we measure our goals, it is often an excruciating process of searching our hearts to find something we are truly passionate about. Initially it may be a little bit depressing to be fully aware of how low our enthusiasm might be for a particular task, but balancing our energy and re-measuring seems to enhance and reinforce the improvements we experience, and make our tasks more effortless and joyful.

Measuring the Attractor Value

In Touch for Health, when we balance energy, we improve the equilibrium of the person among their various muscles, meridians, etc. We also improve the harmonious balance between the individual and the environment- the universe. We can use muscle-testing to measure our "attractor value" - the degree to which we are in tune with the context of our lives, and in balance within our surroundings. This is the kind of energetic state that naturally attracts into our lives those people and activities that allow us to reach our goals. In contrast, we can also have an energetic state that seems to repel people, or prevent us from getting what we want in life. This is something we can add to our usual goal balancing, so once you have done your usual pretests, found a goal and rated it on a subjective analog scale (1-10), follow this procedure:

1. Test an IM while making 4 declarative statements about the goal:
a. First, state the goal as an affirmative present time statement., then rephrase the goal slightly in the following ways:
b. I will …
c. I want to …
d. I choose to ….

2. If there is any inhibition of a test muscle on one or more of these statements, we say that there is some stress in the system related to the goal.

3. Test an IM while Making the statement "I have an attractor value of (a number between 1 and 1000 -.a thousand being the best) or higher. Unless your value is lower than your estimate, the IM will remain strong until you reach a maximum number- your attractor value. If your first estimate causes an IM change, keep lowering your estimate until you find the maximum number for which the IM locks. You can use ranges, like "between 500 and 600" to get into the ballpark, and keep narrowing the range until you find a precise maximum number, like 547) Make a note of your number before balancing, and be sure to recheck after balancing.

7. TEST THE SUPRASPINATUS

Stress on Supraspinatus indicates it's something you can probably benefit from working on. If the Supraspinatus doesn't indicate stress, then you are probably in balance for that goal at that moment in the way that you are stating the thought. Restating your goal, or imagining another desired outcome of your goal will often show the imbalances related to your goal. Look at it from another angle or perspective. We are all very well trained in adapting and coping and are generally not in the habit of "revealing our weak spots", especially verbally. It really isn't surprising that perhaps we manage to find a way of phrasing a goal that we can already feel balanced about.

Do Something:

We can use this goal setting process with any energy balancing or therapeutic modality. We use TFH to integrate the mental/emotional process of goal setting with the postural, muscular, neurological, energetic work of muscle testing, touching reflexes and contemplating the 5 Element Metaphors. Using goals and addressing all of the Soul "parts" in our muscle testing, we can ask what do we imagine is blocking our energy when we have an inhibited muscle in the assessment. We can suggest what functions are controlled by the meridian and what emotions are associated with the meridian. If it brings an awareness to the mind, if emotions are evoked, healing can more easily take place because we are involving more of the whole person in the process.

Thinking about the metaphors corresponding to the muscles which test weak and relating these concepts to your goal can often provide surprising insights as well as release stress and balance your energy around these issues.

NOTICE CHANGE

Take some time to ***put your experience into words***.
Verbalize the positive changes in how you are thinking and feeling (physically, emotionally, mentally and spiritually). Clarify your words by quantifying them. Make a new assessment on an analog scale and re-check your Attractor Value. Be sure that you Re-test to affirm your energy balance in the whole Soul. Reinforce your experience of positive change by listening to your partner's observations and confirm those observations that are true for you.

Reassess your goal to see how far you've come, what parts of your goal have been transformed through the goal setting and energy balancing process.

Decide and make note of the next time/schedule for reassessing your goal(s), reassessing your Soul, and doing something to balance your energies.

The biofeedback mechanism of manual muscle testing is highly effective for re-enforcing both mental and physical awareness of change in the balance of the Soul's energy. The fact that an energy balancing intervention results in the facilitation of "weak" muscles is a powerful positive reinforcement. It's helpful to put this reinforcement into words, and to quantify it by making a new assessment on an analog scale. The healing system is coordinated and integrated. The comparisons that you make between where you were and where you are now , and between where you are now and where you want to be provide valuable information to the healing, welling system of the whole Soul and help to create the experience of life that you desire.

SUCCESS IS GETTING WHAT YOU WANT
HAPPINESS IS WANTING WHAT YOU GET

Goal Protocol ~ Comments

A Protocol for Fix-As-You-Go Balancing
Using Metaphors as a Primary Intervention

1. Establish a goal that you feel enthusiastic about and you believe is possible.

2. Do any pretests that you normally do

3. Check the Central and Governing meridians, and balance any meridian found inhibited using the usual reflexes (i.e. spinal reflex if bilateral weakness is found, then NL, NV, meridians, etc. or use circuit location if you prefer)

AND--- as you use the touch reflex, refer to the metaphors for the Central and Governing meridians.
Example, Central: "What subtle, small thing do you need to let go of?" Example, Governing: "What burden do you need to release?"

4. Check the rest of the meridians and balance any found inhibited using the following guidelines for using metaphors :

   4a. Before using any touch reflexes, offer the word or concept of each metaphor and see what idea or meaning it suggests to the person being balanced in the context of his or her life/goals.

   4b. Present the metaphors as only possibly meaningful. Clarify your own understanding of the traditional meaning of the metaphor, or of your interpretation in this context only to "prime the pump" and get ideas flowing, rather than dictate meaning.

   4c. It may be fruitful to talk over all of the metaphors if it feels appropriate for both people, but it isn't necessary to talk about all of them. Sometimes just one metaphor "rings the bell".

Fix as you go Balancing

4d. Recheck the muscle to confirm that it is now strong. If the muscle has remained inhibited, see if contemplating additional related metaphors rings a bell for the person. Finally, if you've exhausted the metaphors and the muscle is still weak, continue with the touch reflexes. Do this with each of the muscles representing the meridians until no further imbalances are indicated by muscle tests.

5. Reassess your goal and how you are feeling, noting whether any of the metaphors will be valuable for you to hold in mind to enhance your ongoing awareness, dynamism, and balance.

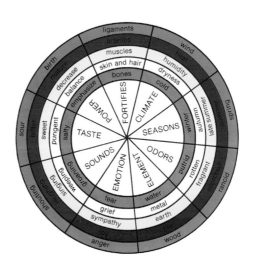

Fix as you go Balancing

A Protocol for Assessment Balancing
Using Metaphors as a Primary Intervention

1. Set a goal that you're enthusiastic about and believe is possible.

2. Do any pretests that you normally do.

3. Check the Central and Governing meridians, and balance any meridian found inhibited using the usual reflexes (i.e. spinal reflex if bilateral weakness is found, then NL, NV, meridians, etc. or use circuit location if you prefer)

AND--- as you use the touch reflex, refer to the metaphors for the Central and Governing meridians.
Example, Central: "What subtle, small thing do you need to let go of?" Example, Governing: "What burden do you need to release?"

4. Check the rest of the indicators for the remaining meridians, recording results on the 5-Element diagram, and/or the Midday Midnight/ 24 Hour "Wheel".

   (4b. If you are going to check for over-energy, use the Alarm Points or Pulse Points to establish over-energy pattern.)

5. Assess the best place to begin balancing according to the 5-Element or "wheel" rules. (see notes starting on page 70)

6. Once you've chosen the appropriate meridian to start with, refer to the metaphors associated with the muscle/meridian/element, following these guidelines:

   6a. Offer the word or Concept of each metaphor and see what idea or meaning it suggests to the person being balanced in the context of his or her life/goals.

6b. Present the metaphors as only possibly meaningful. Clarify your own understanding of the traditional meaning of the metaphor, or of your interpretation in this context only to "prime the pump" and get ideas flowing, rather than dictate meaning.

6c. It may be fruitful to talk over all of the metaphors if it feels appropriate for both people, but it isn't necessary to talk about all of them. Sometimes just one metaphor "rings the bell".

6d. Recheck the muscle to confirm that it is now strong. If the muscle has remained inhibited, see if contemplating additional related metaphors rings a bell for the person. Finally, if you've exhausted the metaphors and the muscle is still weak, continue with the touch reflexes.

7. After correction, recheck all (under-energy) muscles to confirm that they are now facilitated. Correct any that may have remained inhibited, repeating steps 6a-6d.

(7b. If you have checked over-energy, recheck ALL alarm points- all should now be clear. Use the acupressure holding points for sedation of any over-energy that may have remained.)

8. Reassess your goal and how you are feeling, noting whether any of the metaphors will be valuable for you to hold in mind to enhance your ongoing awareness, dynamism, and balance.

Assessment Balancing

Testimonials
Touch for Health helps with confidence in your professional and your personal life.

TFH has rejuvenated my excitement about chiropractic. TFH helps me do muscle testing more quickly in a repeatable fashion.
— **Chin Chow, DC**

I came to get an education and I left with a "new found passion" - a renewed life as a doctor towards treating patients again. Not only did I find a lost part of myself but I discovered a new and wonderful way to take better care of my patients and myself!!
— **Paul Lance Thomas, DC**

TFH inspires me to continue working towards holistic functional integration-living what I love to do and loving how I am living. Thank you **x** infinity.
— **Caroline Hobbson, DC**

After more than 600 hours of Applied Kinesiology, this course has shown me new ways to use the tools I already know and a few new handy tools.
— **Robert Haberkorn, DC**

I have greater confidence in myself as a doctor dealing with all aspects of health. TFH is a truly holistic approach to healing.
— **Rodney Ruge, DC**

Testimonials

68

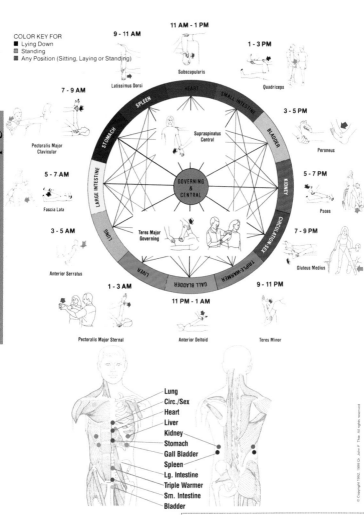

24 HOUR LAW Reference page

24 HOUR LAW

CUT ALONG DOTTED LINE TO CREATE TABS

About the 24-Hour Meridian Cycle
(Meridian Massage/ Meridian Dance)

Since the meridian flow is actually one continuous unbroken flow, the energy flows in one definite direction, and from one meridian to another in a well-determined order. Since there is no beginning and no end to this flow, we represent the order of the meridians as a wheel.

The two midline systems are Central and Governing. Central meridian flows from the pubic bone up the center of the body to the lower lip. Governing flows up from the tailbone up the spine, over the top of the head to the upper lip. These do not ebb and flow at set points on the twenty-four hour clock as do the other 12 meridians. They are storage vessels for the meridian energies and deal with excess or used energy entering and leaving the body.

As we go around this wheel, following the meridian lines, the flow follows this order on the body:
from torso to fingertip, along the inside ("yinside") of the arm-yin.
from fingertip to face, along the outside/back of the arm-yang.
from face to feet, along the outside of the leg-yang.
from feet to torso, along the inside of the leg-yin.

We go through this four step process three times to cover the twelve major meridians. Running the meridians with the hands can be a quick energizing massage. Complete the massage by running the central and governing meridians, which run directly up the back and the front of the body to the upper and lower lip. When we do this with a partner, tracing each other, or in a group, each tracing our own meridians, we call it the *Meridian Dance*.

Notes on Energy Pattern Assessment

The 24-hour graphic illustrates 4 different cycles/relationships among the meridians and the Five Element graphic illustrates an additional 2 cycles. The muscle-test thumbnails for the Central (Supraspinatus) and Governing (Teres Major) meridians are shown in the center of the wheel, since they function more as storage vessels related to all of the meridians, rather than part of the 24-hour cycle. The muscle-test thumbnails of the primary tests for other 12 meridians are shown on the outside of the wheel . They are color-coded: red for tests which are the same sitting, standing, or lying down, blue for standing tests, black for lying down tests. Above each thumbnail is the spinal reflex associated with the given muscle and the peak energy period for the given meridian. At the bottom of the page is a figure illustrating the Alarm Points, which we can used to check for over-energy, see further explanation below.

Energy Patterns in the 24-hour Graphic:
1. "Beaver Dam"

A block in the 24-hour meridian cycle is indicated by three or more consecutive meridians inhibited in a clockwise direction. We call this a "beaver dam" because clearing the block "upstream" in the cycle will generally clear all the subsequent blocks following in the 24-hour cycle. Consider the metaphors and use the balancing points related to the first meridian in a clockwise direction.

If you check for over-energy, start with the first under-energy, FOLLOWING AN OVER-ENERGY meridian in clockwise order.

2. Triangles

There are 3 yin and 3 yang meridians which travel in the same direction on the arms and legs. These are represented by blue triangles on the 24-hour graphic, If 2 or 3 meridians are inhibited, look at the metaphors of the first imbalance, closest to time of day.

If you check for over-energy, look for one over energy and two under energy meridians. Start with the first under-energy, following an over-energy meridian in clockwise order.

3. Squares

The meridians travel the entire body 3 times, head to foot, foot to trunk, trunk to hands, and hands to head. Each circuit of the body is represented on the graphic by a square of 4 meridians. If three 3 or 4 meridians on a square are inhibited, look at the metaphors of the first imbalance, closest to time of day.

If you check for over-energy, look for one over-energy and three under-energy meridians (more than one over-energy meridian in a square is considered random, and so not a square pattern). Start with the first under-energy, following an over-energy meridian in clockwise order.

In addition, each square has a common function among its four related meridians. The Square (or circuit) containing Stomach, Liver, Circulation/Sex and Small Intestine relates to metabolic, anabolic, and catabolic functions. The Square containing Spleen, Triple Warmer, Lung and Bladder has a common Immune Function. The square for Heart, Gall Bladder, Kidney, and Large Intestine has a common association with spiritual/emotional functions.

If you have a "square" imbalance, you might consider these functions as a possible symbol for what is going on in your life, in addition to the 5-Element, Meridian, and Muscle Metaphors.

4. Spokes

Meridians 12 hours apart in the 24-hour cycle are related because one is at its highest flow while the other is at its lowest ebb. These are illustrated by spokes on the wheel. If both are inhibited, start with the meridian closest to the time of day.

If you check for over-energy, look for one over-energy and the other under-energy. Start with the under-energy meridian.

24 HOUR Pattern Assessment

ALARM POINTS
Locations of Alarm Points
Lung: Bilaterally, at junction of shoulder and chest

Circulation Sex: Midline, on the sternum at the level of the nipples

Heart: Midline, at the end of the breast bone on the zyphoid process

Stomach: Midline, 1/2 way between heart alarm point and navel

Large Intestine: Bilaterally, 1 1/2 body inches beside the navel

Triple Warmer: Midline, 2 - 3 body inches below the navel

Small Intestine: Midline, 2 - 3 body inches below triple warmer

Bladder: Midline, just above of the pubic bone

Liver: Bilaterally, below the nipples at the 7th and 8th rib space

Gall Bladder: Bilaterally, on the costal border at the level of 9th rib

Spleen: Bilaterally, at the tip of the 11th rib (side seam of body)

Kidney: Bilaterally, at the tip of the 12th rib

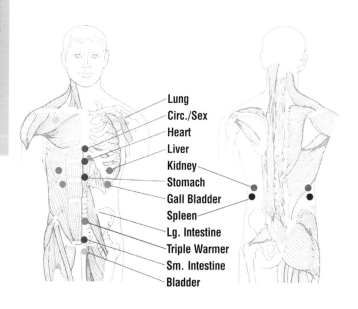

Lung
Circ./Sex
Heart
Liver
Kidney
Stomach
Gall Bladder
Spleen
Lg. Intestine
Triple Warmer
Sm. Intestine
Bladder

ALARM POINTS

About Alarm Points

Sometimes a muscle that tests somewhat weak at first seems to get even weaker as you work with the spinal reflexes, neurolymphatic points, neurovascular points, etc. One possibility is that the meridian involved already may be over-energized. Weak muscle tests usually mean the meridian needs stimulation, but an over-energized meridian can 'pop the circuit' and make its associated muscle weak. Naturally, if it is already overloaded, any further stimulation you give it, the more imbalance is being created.

To see if a meridian is over-energized, first find and test a strong Indicator Muscle (IM). Lightly touch the 'alarm point' associated with the meridian and test the IM. If the IM goes weak when you re-test while holding the 'alarm point,' over-energy is indicated. To make the correction, find the **acupressure holding points** on the reference page for the associated meridian/muscle. Locate the sedation points. Hold them lightly. Now re-test, touching the 'alarm point' and then immediately re-test the weak muscle. Both should test strong.

Also, use the Alarm points to check each meridian for over-energy when doing an assessment balance.

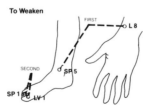

Acupressure Holding Points

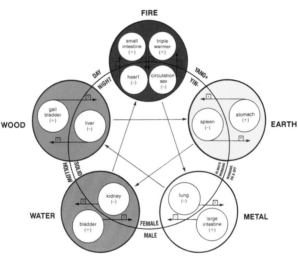

FIRE

small intestine (+)   triple warmer (+)

heart (−)   circulation sex (−)

DAY / NIGHT

YANG+ / YIN−

WOOD

gall bladder (+)   liver (−)

HOLLOW / SOLID

EARTH

spleen (−)   stomach (+)

ALWAYS WORKING / TURNING ON & OFF

MOTION

WATER

kidney (−)   bladder (+)

FEMALE / MALE

METAL

lung (−)   large intestine (+)

PULSE CHECK

LEFT HAND

LIGHT TOUCH
● Small Intestine
● Gall Bladder
● Bladder

DEEP TOUCH
● Heart
● Liver
● Kidneys

RIGHT HAND

LIGHT TOUCH
● Large Intestine
● Stomach
● Triple Warmer

DEEP TOUCH
● Lung
● Spleen
● Circulation -sex

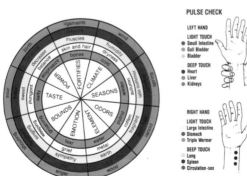

5 ELEMENTS

About the 5 Element Cycles

This traditional Chinese paradigm represents all aspects of the universe and natural cycles of the earth (rather than the chemical elements of Western science). As a product of folklore, it is a metaphor portraying immutable truths. As such it covers the phases of the life cycle.

From the birth phase came WOOD
The surging upwards phase produced FIRE
In its mature adult stage was EARTH
In the decay phase, METAL
In its death/rebirth phase, WATER

Two Energy Cycles
Two separate cycles of energy interact to keep the balance of all things in the universe.

The SHEN(G) cycle is the generating and nurturing cycle, which moves consecutively in a clockwise fashion through the elements.

In so doing, the "mother" element is said to create and nurture the "daughter" element. For example, Wood is said to be the mother of Fire because it feeds it, Fire is the mother of Earth creating it from its ashes, Earth gives up its ores to create Metal, Metal produces the Water, and Water nurtures the Wood

The other energy cycle is the KO or control cycle in which each element has a controlling influence over the second element from it, in the clockwise cycle. This is represented by a star pattern on the graphic. Therefore, Wood is called the "grandmother" of Earth and controls it by penetrating it, Earth controls Water by containing it, Water controls Fire by dowsing it, Fire controls Metal by melting it, and Metal controls Wood by chopping it.

Other qualities are shown in the elements e.g. emotions, sounds and colors, tastes and smells, and the seasons. There is also a representation of the yin and yang meridian energy of the body. All of these characteristics are meaningful to those trained in Traditional Chinese medicine. For example, the experienced Chinese physician would look for imbalances in these qualities, noticing if the person had a specific hue to their complexion, a particular resonance to their voice, a preference or dislike for the seasons, tastes, and so on.

In our two dimensional model, one energy cycle is superimposed upon the other, and it should be remembered that each cycle affects the Five Elements in their entirety. Surplus energy moves around the Five Elements in a clockwise direction and takes the shortest route. It will use either cycle to do this, shunting energy through the meridian system.

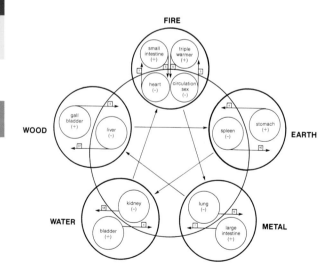

5-Element Assessment

A. Do the usual Pre-tests and set a goal.

B. Do a 14 or more muscle assessment
(correct Central and Governing first.)

C. Simple Model:

1. Look for a series of meridian imbalances going in a clockwise direction using either Shen or Ko cycles. Correct the first unlocked muscle in the series- *but always prefer to start with a YIN meridian, these are the meridians on the inside of the circle* (Begin with Yin, Yin is in).

C. *Over Energy Model:*

1. Check ALARM POINTS to establish over energy pattern. Use a light touch on alarm points.

2. Start with the FIRST YIN UNDER-ENERGY AFTER ANY OVER-ENERGY(going in a clockwise direction using either Shen or Ko cycle).

3. You may also use Circuit Locating with the spinal reflex, neurolymphatics, etc. to confirm the appropriate meridian fto start with. Continue to circuit locate the reflex points and retest other under energy muscles. These should now lock, showing that your key reflex point will move energy to balance all other meridians. Make the correction and Challenge in the usual way.

D. After correction, recheck all under energy muscles to confirm that they are now locked, (and recheck all Alarm Points - all should now be clear.)

E. Recheck goal statement - should now test clear. If the goal still inhibits the IM, use E.S.R to clear. Reassess goal on an analog scale and reassess how you are feeling.

5-Element Assessment

Pulse Test

Taken from the Chinese pulse diagnosis, the pulse check allows us to monitor excess energy in the meridians. In TFH we assess mainly "under-energy" as indicated by a muscle unlocking. But sometimes the muscle unlocks because of "over-energy". If we are assessing the energy in all of the muscles/meridians before making any correction, we can also check for any over-energy to help decide the best place to start. We can check for over-energy in the following way:

1. Do the usual pre-checks. Hold the left wrist in the right hand and muscle test the opposite arm as an IM, or have the person to place the back of their left wrist in their right palm with the right index, middle and ring fingers positioned immediately below the wrist crease as shown in the diagram on page 79 and on the 5-Element Reference Page. Use a light touch to represent the energy of the three yang meridians.

2. If the person is holding his or her own wrist, you can use a leg indicator muscle to test. If there is a change in IM, test each finger separately to determine the yang meridian involved.

3. Repeat the original test with three fingers, using deep pressure, representing the yin meridians.

4. Now go to the opposite wrist and test in the same way.

Balance:

For each over-energized meridian, use the acupressure holding points for sedation to balance the meridian's energy. Recheck each pulse point that weakened the indicator muscle. All should now be strong, showing the person is balanced.

NOTE: The 5-Element Reference Page also contains the "pie" figure of the traditional 5-Element Metaphors. This will give you quick reference to the metaphors associated with a given element. Example questions for each element are provided in subsequent sections.

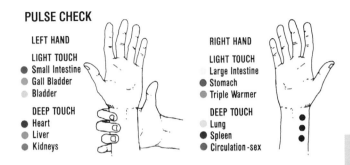

PULSE CHECK

LEFT HAND

LIGHT TOUCH
● Small Intestine
● Gall Bladder
● Bladder

DEEP TOUCH
● Heart
● Liver
● Kidneys

RIGHT HAND

LIGHT TOUCH
○ Large Intestine
● Stomach
● Triple Warmer

DEEP TOUCH
○ Lung
● Spleen
● Circulation-sex

Why 2 assessment models?

Why only two TFH models of assessment?

In every scientific work there is the science part-- empirical or experimental evidence that a technique is effective for the desired outcome, and there is an art/spirit part-- the subtle, personal differences which work best for the individuals involved, whether they adhere to the traditional or prescribed methods or not.

No Single Right Way

Touch for Health is both a science and an art. We show two models of assessment balancing (simple, and over-energy) because these models are ones that have a long history and tradition of use and are good examples of what has worked for a lot of people. At the same time, providing 2 models helps us to see that there is not only one right way of doing things in Touch for Health.

Everyone who uses the methods brings with them knowledge as well as their personal intuition and insight. Everyone who practices Touch for Health eventually finds their own particular way to do each technique that is most effective in helping start the natural healing system in each person in the encounter. This is OK and part of the art and spirit of TFH.

The important thing to remember is that when using a particular model you need to know the assumptions of the model. You cannot know or perceive everything at any one time so we develop models that simplify our experience for specific purposes. As long as you recognize the limitations of a model-- the assumptions and limited purpose of the model-- we can get the best results, and recognize when we need to expand our model, or switch models entirely.

Why 2 assessment models?

In the simple assessment model we balance the energy in the central and governing meridians first which allows used or excess energy to leave the body with the breath. We then assume that we have cleared any over-energy and that all the other meridian energy blocks will show as under energy most of the time, and correct based on under energy. However, if a muscle doesn't get facilitated by touching the reflex points but actually seems to get more inhibited, then we check for an over-energy in that meridian. We use the associated Alarm Point, or check the Pulse Points, and correct the over-energy using the Acupressure Holding Points. We can also check for any residual over-energy after balancing the 14 meridians and correct with the AHP's.

In the over-energy model we do not make any assumption about over-energy. We check all the meridians for under energy, as indicated by unlocking muscles, and then and we check for over-energy as indicated by the alarm points or the pulse points. The assessment is then made on the pattern of over and under-energy as a whole.

Some people prefer the slightly more sophisticated method of the over-energy model, while others prefer to **KISS** (Keep It Simple, Sweetheart)

REFERENCE

PAGE NO.	CHART SECTION	MUSCLE	RELATED ORGAN	MERIDIAN	TIME	TFH BOOK PAGE/MUSCLE TEST NUMBER
5	4	Abdominals	Small Intestine	Small Intestine	2 PM	57
8	7	Adductors	Sex	Circulation-Sex	8 PM	73
10	9	Ant. Deltoid	Gall Bladder	Gall Bladder	12 Mid.	89
2	1	Ant. Neck Flexors	Sinuses	Stomach	8 AM	41
12	11	Ant. Serratus	Lungs	Lung	4 AM	97
	5	Ant. Tibial	Bladder	Bladder	4 PM	63
2	1	Brachioradialis	Stomach	Stomach	8 AM	43
12	11	Coracobrachialis	Lungs	Lung	4 AM	99
12	11	Deltoids	Lungs	Lung	4 AM	101
12	11	Diaphragm	Lungs	Lung	4 AM	103
13	12	Fascia Lata	Large Intestine	Large Intestine	6 AM	105
9	8	Gastrocnemius	Adrenals	Triple-Warmer	10 PM	87
8	7	Gluteus Maximus	Sex	Circulation-Sex	8 PM	77
8	7	Gluteus Medius	Sex	Circulation-Sex	8 PM	71
9	8	Gracilis	Adrenals	Triple-Warmer	10 PM	83
13	12	Hamstrings	Large Intestine	Large Intestine	6 AM	107
7	6	Iliacus	Ileo-Cecal Valve	Kidney	6 PM	69
3	2	Latissimus Dorsi	Pancreas	Spleen	10 AM	45
2	1	Levator Scapulae	Stomach	Stomach	8 AM	39
3	2	Lower Trapezius	Spleen	Spleen	10 AM	47
3	2	Middle Trapezius	Spleen	Spleen	10 AM	47
3	2	Opponens Pol. Longus	Spleen	Spleen	10 AM	49
2	1	Pectoralis Maj. Clav.	Stomach	Stomach	8 AM	37
11	10	Pectoralis Maj. Sternal	Liver	Liver	2 AM	93
	5	Peroneus	Bladder	Bladder	4 PM	59
8	7	Piriformis	Sex	Circulation-Sex	8 PM	75
10	9	Popliteus	Gall Bladder	Gall Bladder	12 Mid.	91
2	1	Post. Neck Extensors	Sinuses	Stomach	8 AM	41
	5	Post. Tibial	Bladder	Bladder	4 PM	63
7	6	Psoas	Kidneys	Kidney	6 PM	65
13	12	Quadratus Lumborum	Spine	Large Intestine	6 AM	109
5	4	Quadriceps	Small Intestine	Small Intestine	2 PM	55
11	10	Rhomboids	Liver	Liver	2 AM	95
	5	Sacrospinalis	Bladder	Bladder	4 PM	61
9	8	Sartorius	Adrenals	Triple-Warmer	10 PM	81
9	8	Soleus	Adrenals	Triple-Warmer	10 PM	85
4	3	Subscapularis	Heart	Heart	12 Noon	53
1	13	Supraspinatus	Brain	Central	8 PM	33
1	13	Teres Major	Spine	Governing	12 Noon	35
9	8	Teres Minor	Thyroid	Triple-Warmer	10 PM	79
3	2	Triceps	Pancreas	Spleen	10 AM	51
7	6	Upper Trapezius	Eyes & Ears	Kidney	6 PM	67

Muscle/Meridian REFERENCE

About the Muscle/Meridian REFERENCE Page

This page lists all 42 TFH muscles in alphabetical order. The corresponding organs/meridians are listed as well as reference page/section numbers for this Metaphor Pocketbook, the TFH Reference Chart (The same reference info. as in the Reference Folio, but in a wall chart form), and the TFH manual.

• The first column lists the "page numbers" of the reference pages in the Pocketbook, and are color coded to match the colored tabs at the bottom of each reference page. These are the colors from ancient Chinese tradition related to the meridians in the 24 hour cycle as compared to the colors of the five elements.

• The second column lists the corresponding sections in the TFH Reference wall chart.

• The third column lists the 42 TFH muscles in alphabetical order.

• The fourth column lists the related physiological organ. However, in TFH we are making no inference as to the condition of the organ itself, but rather think of the function of the organ as a metaphor for that kind of function in the whole person and in their life.

• The fifth column lists the related Chi energy meridian. We are mainly interested in the balance of energy among all the meridians, and meridian function as a metaphor for function of the whole person.

• The sixth column lists the time of day that the meridian is most active. (The opposite time of day, 12 midnight instead of 12 noon, for example, would be its lowest ebb)

• The seventh column lists the corresponding page in the TFH manual

• The last column is again color coded to match the colored tabs at the bottom of each reference page which also correspond to the traditional 24-hr cycle of the meridians.

About the Touch for Health Metaphors

The mental exercise of contemplating the metaphors increases parallel processing in diverse areas of the brain and the whole Soul, bringing more of our innate resources to bear in balancing our energies for our unique purposes. Just thinking or talking about the metaphor often balances the energy in all of the meridians as indicated by muscle testing. But thinking about the metaphors also provides all kinds of insights and new perspectives for our life experience.

When we use the word "metaphor", we use it in its broadest sense. We suggest symbolic pictures or actions, figurative or literal similarities, parallels, corollaries etc. We are looking for any imagery that vividly illustrates or represents some significant aspect of your life. This is largely a creative/associative activity. It may help give you specific conscious insight into your personal life issues, or it may simply help to "get the juices flowing".

The metaphors that correspond to the meridian or muscle imbalance may not apply for your particular goal. They are presented as possibly meaningful, but are not necessarily applicable at a particular moment for a particular person. It is for the person seeking help to decide if the metaphors make sense to them, or helps them have meaning in their lives.

See if any of the metaphors fit your life now, or might relate to some event in the past, or are symbolic of your direction for the future. Start with the basic metaphor and see if it "rings a bell". If the suggested metaphor fits, great. If another idea jumps to mind, consider that to be more significant. If the metaphor doesn't fit, and nothing comes to mind, then you might just move on. Or perhaps there is a particular emotion you are feeling when you think of the metaphor. Try to verbalize it, to express it, or simply to be aware of it.

About TFH Metaphors

When we leave ourselves open to imagination, free association and non-sequitur responses to the metaphors, we often find strong emotions bubbling up. These may be emotions that have been dismissed or diverted during the day, or repressed over long periods of time. Emotions have a major physical component, and if we can find a safe space to express and release our emotions, we often find it a great physical relief.

We need to remember that people have hard wired into their Souls the imperatives for survival: hunger, sexual desire, fear, avoidance of pain etc. The emotions, anger, joy, sympathy, grief, fear, etc. are there to mobilize our Soul, our body-mind-spirit, to deal with our survival needs. Denying our emotions and feelings may be literally necessary for survival or to deal with a difficult situation. But habitual or permanent suppression of our emotions can block the flow of energy in the Soul, the whole person, and keep us from utilizing our talents to the fullest, and discovering our unique mission in life. Consider that you may want to allow yourself to experience the emotions that come out when you are balancing your energy and thinking of the metaphors. Be sure that the authority remains with the person being balanced so that if emotions become overwhelming, they can choose to stop and "think of fresh bread" or some other neutral, calming image.

The Five Element Metaphors

In TFH we assume that the 5000-year-old Chinese Five Element Metaphors are pictorial or symbolic and thus can have many interpretations. The eleven aspects of each of the elements will be best understood if the words are thought of as pictures that are brought to mind when the words are spoken. We store nearly all of our knowledge and memory in sensory images, which relate to our five senses, our emotions, intuition, and our sense of importance or meaning. The Five Element metaphors are used to elicit associations with images, ideas, sensations and feelings that are meaningful in the context of your life and your current goals.

The Chinese word-picture symbol for "element" might more accurately be translated as "phase". The original pictograph for "xing" means to walk, to move. It suggests action, process and change. Thus, the Five Elements represent the simultaneous processes that are always occurring and counter-balancing each other. These five processes also intertwine as phases within a variety of cycles. The phases can be related to long cycles such as the seasons of the year or the phases of a human life cycle, or to shorter cycles such as the 24 hour cycle of the day and night or the life cycles of individual cells.

In the Chinese energetic system, there is an emphasis on context and pattern rather than one to one causation. In the West, we tend to seek to dissect a problem, to reduce it to the one cause and the one cure. We attempt to reduce the issue to a single meaning, a named disease that can be killed, or managed. The Traditional healer in China gathers signs and symptoms until a whole picture of the person emerges with many layers of interrelated meanings. The Eastern approach is person centered. Humans are seen as body-mind-spirit entities with aspects which manifest as more physical, mental or spiritual, but are never only one, taking into account an individual's context and purposes, at a particular moment in time.

In TFH, when we are assessing energy, we CAN be analytical, find a dominant imbalance and perhaps pinpoint the one most logical place to start balancing, often using only one correction and finding all of the muscles subsequently facilitated. We might be able to prioritize a single key metaphor and balance the energy with that one idea. Certainly there will be times when this kind of efficiency is precisely what we want, but in general our approach is to be aware of as many factors as possible. At any time we may have more than one dominant imbalance. For each different issue or goal we usually see a different pattern of imbalances. Layering of information gives us a whole picture of a person assembled within the context of a whole life.

The explanations and questions provided in this Pocketbook are my own creative interpretation of the Five Element metaphors, based some on the traditional concepts of the symbols and some on my own more western associations. You will probably benefit more from your own reactions to the word/picture metaphors, and contemplating whatever "comes to you" or "pops into your head", than by forcing any "correct" interpretation, according to me or to tradition. Many of my ideas may very well be "wrong" in terms of traditional Chinese Medicine, and those for whom these cultural meanings are familiar can simply disregard my mistakes. But I suggest that you first see what the symbols elicit in you, and what they tell you about yourself. Refer to my explanations and questions as an example of how you might derive meaning from the metaphors. Finally, you might do some of your own research into the original traditional texts as a further resource for your own insight, rather than as an authority which dictates the "correct" interpretation.

In TFH we use ten traditional metaphors associated with each of the Five Elements. I have integrated an 11th metaphor cycle from my study of the phases of cognitive and philosophical development, which I call the Faith/Worldview Metaphor Cycle. The phases of human development of beliefs and world-views correspond to a linear model of mental capacity for certain modes of thinking (cognitive development) as well as a progression through stages of spiritual or philosophical concepts. However, I also believe that each individual may cycle through these perspectives throughout their life and in relation to different goals or issues.

Faith/Worldview Metaphor Cycle
Each of us uses a variety of different models of reality to make sense of our experience, to make decisions, to improve performance and have more personal bests. Each of these models entails certain assumptions and ideas that we believe to be true, even though we may not be conscious of these beliefs. We may not recognize our faith in the assumptions of our own worldview as faith. We might want to simply call it "Reality". We might just say, "that's just how life is."

About TFH Metaphors

When I use the word Faith I want to define it as the process by which we actively construct our personal world-view, the set of beliefs which allow each of us to have meaning in our lived lives and make conscious decisions.

Our beliefs constitute our holistic, largely unconscious and unarticulated conception of our experience of life, and the way the world works-- what is really real, and what laws govern what is possible. For me, Faith is the active spiritual element in our walk of consciously striving to discover and be aware of the truest, deepest, most powerful meaning in our lives and to develop our belief, actions, and way of being to be in harmony with these truths. This can take the form of a personal relationship as in prayer with God or Jesus. Our beliefs/worldview and Faith are the fundamental force that shapes our experience and perception, our priorities and passions. It tends to progress in stages through the life span, but it is also ever-changing, evolving, and cycling through different phases. Our beliefs and faith may be in different phases for different issues or aspects of our life. Contemplating an open system of metaphors that have been used for 5000 years, we can gain insight into and awareness of our own beliefs in general, and in relation to specific life issues and goals.

The Organ Function Metaphors

It should be noted that the Chinese conceptions of the Organ Functions differ significantly from the traditional western medical conception of the functions of the actual physical organs. In traditional Chinese philosophy, Organs are seen as metaphors, symbolic representations of FUNCTIONS. It is the Organ Function that is said to create the physical organ rather than the physical structure dictating the function. Physical organs are a phenomenon of, or expressions of Organ Functions, not mechanistic structures that can be fully understood through anatomical dissection. The actual mechanism will never be fully understood, but can be appreciated through a holistic conception of the Organ Function metaphor.

About TFH Metaphors

In TFH we are comfortable with imprecise, or subjective understanding because we only use SAFE energy balancing reflexes, and emphasize that each person must be aware of themselves, and take responsibility to avail themselves of professional healers when they find that they need more help than TFH can provide. We do TFH as a daily hygiene, not as a medical treatment of a disease. We benefit from the subjective, imprecise nature of the metaphors, because each individual is unique, and so requires a unique interpretation of the metaphor related to their life experience. There is no fixed, "correct" answer, only answers that ring true for the person at the moment.

Organ functions are Global. They take place in the whole person and in every cell. Each cell in the human being has all the functions of the 5 Elements. Physical malfunction of a specific organ may not correspond to energy imbalance of the Organ Function in the whole Soul. Likewise, energy imbalance of an Organ Function may not be reflected in the physical organ. This would mean that you could have a malfunction or injury in the foot that results in an imbalance in the energy of the Liver Function. This does not indicate that injury to the foot has caused direct damage to the liver, but rather that the Liver Functions of the cells of the foot are communicating a subtle energy block that may be alleviated using the reflexes, or the metaphors of the Liver Functions.

My experience over the many years I have been using and developing the TFH system has shown me that even serious pathology of an organ will often not show a muscle indicator inhibition or over energy for the associated meridian. The cells making up that physical organ can have other meridian energy imbalances blocking the healing energy flow and allowing pathology of the organ. In using TFH we are more interested in helping the person select and obtain personal goals than in working with named diseases, pathologies or injuries directly. You may be able to reach your goal without having a disappearance of the pathology, or you may have a balancing of energy which will in turn allow the internal healing system to function and resolve the pathology. Think of the Organ Metaphor not in terms of any discrete physical organ, but in terms of the associated Function as a symbol for what is happening in your life.

If you are aware of a diagnosed pathology of an organ or of any kind, be sure to consult a professional who is qualified to work within the biomedical model of diagnosis and medical treatment. You can use TFH to supplement medical treatment by contemplating what an ailment means in your life, or what the scientific facts symbolize in metaphorical terms. A heart attack, or liver disease or even a sore throat has more than physical meaning. We can use TFH to consider how our knowledge of diagnosed conditions resonates emotionally, spiritually, and symbolically within the whole context of our lives, to alleviate associated stress, and to balance our energy for optimal function of our immune system. In the context of TFH, these metaphors are not taken literally to reflect the clinical status of a physical organ. Rather, we examine the meanings that we attach to the organs and explore how those meanings might also reflect some aspect of our experience of our lives. Some Western physiological conceptions of organ functions are integrated into this discussion as another possible source of meaningful metaphors, rather than as a resource for diagnosing organ based physical conditions.

Muscle Metaphors

Muscles are not used in isolation. For every muscle that contracts, some muscles must relax or be inhibited, some muscles must fix the origin and other muscles must also become active to allow smooth motion in the specific direction desired. The TFH muscle tests utilize a general position that partially isolates a specific muscle, putting other muscles in a less active mode. We will get the best results if we also feel the muscle contracting while the test is being preformed. Try to become aware of the specific muscle as you perform the range of motion. Once you have a conscious and kinetic sense of the range of motion, try to be aware of any thoughts or feelings that come to mind. Think of what kind of action this motion suggests. Does the literal

About TFH Metaphors

activity correspond to your life or your goal? What might the activity symbolize in your life?

Think of what the motion suggests to you. Then, if you need some inspiration, check if the explanation of the muscle action and the sample questions mean something to you. Does anything "pop into your head"? Maybe you can contemplate that, even if it doesn't seem to have any direct, literal relation to the muscle action accept your free association, intuition or subtle internal communication .

The metaphors are mostly used during the energy balancing and might also be referred to when discussing the outcome of the balancing, but after the balancing, our focus is on the specific meanings for the individual person, rather than the metaphors per se. This allows the person being helped to tell his or her story and discover where their passions are and where they are wounded, damaged or in denial.

Learning to use metaphors effectively involves the practice of listening and other communication skills. This may be inter-personal communication, or communication with ourselves, self-awareness. The person seeking help will often have conscious insights related to the metaphors, but also reveal things they might not be aware of through body language, tone of voice, etc. The person acting as helper has an important role in observing responses that the individual may not perceive, may be blind to, or may be in denial about. However, we maintain the self-responsibility model. The helper only offers their observations as possibilities. It is up to the individual to decide on their own meaning.

The helper strives to be attentive. The unique subjective experiences of the individual make the parable, the meaningful story, the life they are living, special and unique. With each metaphor we allow the person to evaluate their subjective balance in relation to the feeling, issue, or story that the metaphor brings to mind. We use TFH to help

About TFH Metaphors

the person become aware of their imbalances, to become more balanced and have the ability to function fully, fulfilling their mission, using their talents and finding their destiny.

Listening to the whole person, we try to hear not only facts, but emotions, incongruities and conflicts, issues of passion and areas of imbalance. We are almost guaranteed success in this exercise if our fundamental effort is to respect the person as important to the whole world by just being who they are at the moment, and to communicate this appreciation. Each person has transcendent value because a power greater than them is working through them. Our efforts at self-awareness and energy balancing are to come into harmony with this great power that we are a part of. We may call this Universal Energy that gives us life and connects us with all creation Chi, Ki, Prana, Holy Spirit, Ruhah, Innate Intelligence, Holy Spirit. For me Jesus the Christ is the personification of that energy in human form. Jesus often spoke in parables, symbolic stories, which have many interpretations according to our needs when we interpret them. We might respect our own symbol-stories as coming from that same source which is also within us, and find direction and meaning in life through their contemplation.

What Does the Metaphor Mean in YOUR Life Right Now? Does that ring a bell? Seem to have some meaning in this context? Make you think of anything? Bring anything to mind? Do you know what that is for you? What could that be an emblem for-- a metaphor symbolizing what?

First look inside yourself for your own association with the metaphor, then consider our interpretations of the traditional Chinese meanings of the symbols and see what response that elicits from you, whether that meaning "fits" in any way. Finally, you might do some further study of the metaphors with the purpose of enriching your own self understanding, rather than forcing your life to fit any "fixed" and "correct" meanings for the metaphors.

CENTRAL: 7-9 PM

RNA

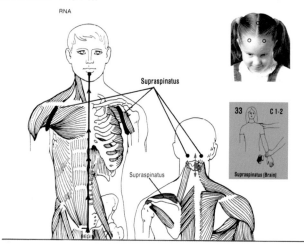

Supraspinatus

Supraspinatus

Supraspinatus

33   C 1-2

Supraspinatus (Brain)

BEGIN

GOVERNING: 11 AM-1 PM

Whole protein

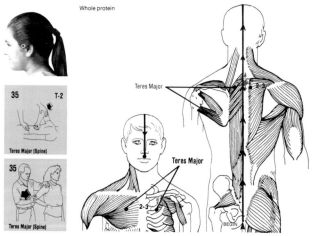

35   T-2

Teres Major (Spine)

35

Teres Major (Spine)

Teres Major

Teres Major

2-3

BEGIN

The Central and Governing Meridians

The Central and Governing meridians relate to the balance of stored energy and the energy leaving the Soul (the whole person). The Governing and Central Meridians are closely associated with the Lung Meridian because they relate to the breath cycle in which subtle energy and air are drawn into and released from the Soul, but they are related to all of the Elements and Organs. The Supraspinatus and Teres Major muscles are used as indicators of the Central and Governing meridians, respectively. These are the first two muscles that are balanced (restored to a facilitated state, testing strong). When the used and stored energy is in balance, then the excess or over energy in any of the other meridians will be more easily brought into balance. This will allow the greatest change and attract those people and things that will allow the fulfillment of our purposes.

Central Meridian Function

The Central Meridian/Conception Vessel is where the used energy is stored prior to being released with the breath on exhaling. All the other meridians have connections with it for releasing the excess and/or used energy. The associated metaphor is of letting go of a previously useful idea, thing, emotion, heuristic truth, worldview etc. It is a short meridian and we use a small muscle (the supraspinatus) as an indicator. Releasing of little, or subtle things can be of great importance to allow new things to occur in your life. Think of exhaling, and letting go of things that once served you, but can now be released. The Central Meridian is related to the Brain Functions of the innate intelligence of the whole Soul in each of the cells and in the overall coordination of your internal wisdom. These are the functions of doing some things automatically (or autonomically), while doing other things consciously; doing more than one thing at a time and changing what you're doing as circumstances change.

What subtle, small thing or idea do you need to release to reach your goal?

Muscle: SUPRASPINATUS

This muscle is a small one related to the shoulder and lifting the arm in a forward position.

Feel this small muscle contracting on top of the shoulder under the neck muscle (under the upper trapezius). This is a subtle feeling. The supraspinatus is a deep muscle. If you feel a muscle contracting or straining elsewhere, check the position of the test or consider the supraspinatus inhibited. If a muscle is not fully facilitated, it may recruit other muscles to compensate.

Test: Position with the straight arm about 30° above the body, slightly to the side with palm facing the groin. Stabilize by placing your other hand on the opposite shoulder. Pressure is on the forearm to push it towards the groin.

What do you need to let go of, particularly some small, subtle thing, that worked for you in the past but is not useful now?

Governing Meridian Function

The Governing meridian is connected with all the other meridians including the Central/Conception vessel. It is a storage vessel for excess or used energy before this energy is released with the breath. Prior to using the other muscles as indicators of imbalances in the Soul (the whole person), it is important to uncover/release this stored energy by considering the burdens that a person is literally or figuratively carrying.

The Governing Meridian is associated with the function of standing and Spine Function. It may also be related to Pineal Function that relates to the day/night cycles of light and darkness.

What transitions are you coping with, or do you need to make? What subtle or dramatic shifts in energy allocation are you making or do you need to make? How do you feel about nighttime vs. daytime? What is your favorite season? What are you carrying

that has become a burden? How can you transition or transform your burden so that it is helpful and not hindering to you?

Muscle: TERES MAJOR—
This is a small muscle of the back of the shoulder, when it isn't working at its optimum (as indicated by testing facilitated /strong) the shoulders tend to slump forward as if you were carrying a weight or heavy burden, literally and metaphorically. This muscle is particularly related to pineal organ function that relates to the day/night cycles of light and darkness.

Feel this small muscle contracting between the top of your arm and the bottom of the shoulder blade.

Test: Position back of hand in the small of the back, bring elbow back as far as is comfortable. Lightly brace the shoulder on the same side. Do not allow the shoulder to drop. Pressure is against the elbow to push it forward.

What burden or weight needs to be removed from your life? How do you envision the burden? Is it a heavy load, a mass of chains, a person? How will you get that off your back? Will you set it down or throw it off? Do you need help to remove your burden? What transitions are you coping with, or do you need to make? What subtle or dramatic shifts in energy allocation are you making or do you need to make? How can you transition or transform your burden so that it is helpful and not hindering to you?

Governing Meridian Metaphors

The Earth Element
Stomach and Spleen Meridians

The Earth Element metaphor corresponds to the ground, the soil, the dirt. The Fire element gives birth to Earth, symbolized by ashes that return to the earth. Earth in turn gives birth to metal, symbolized by the salts, minerals and ores that form in the earth. The Earth Element is controlled by Wood which is symbolized by the roots of trees holding the earth in place. The Earth Element in turn controls water by containing it, giving it form, as in a lake or a river. The Earth Element is associated with the Season of Late Summer, and is said to be a time of Transition not only between summer and autumn, but also between each of the seasons. The Direction associated with the Earth Element is not North, South, East or West, but Center. Thus, the Five Elements are sometimes represented with the Earth Element at the center, with the other four Elements at the cardinal directions.

Do you feel like you have your feet on the ground or do you need to be more grounded and centered? In your current phase of change, do you feel like you have enough roots to nourish your growth and enough stability to give form to your dreams (Water Element)?

The **Color** metaphor associated with the Earth Element is **Yellow.**

What does the color yellow mean to you in your life? Related to your current life goals, what might the color yellow represent?

Yellow might correspond to the **Season** metaphor of the Earth Element which is **Late Summer**, the time of ripening or maturing of the crops and of the early harvest. We might picture fields of crops waiting to be harvested, or the action of harvesting of crops.

Is it time for you to begin to reap the harvest of what you have sewn, or do you need to let things develop a little longer? What in your life needs harvesting, and what needs to be allowed a little more time to mature?

Earth Element Metaphors

The **Climate** metaphor of the Earth Element is **Dampness** or Humidity. We might picture a climate where we perspire without any real exertion. We can think of steam, fog, or mist.

What might humidity, steam, fog or mist symbolize in your life? Do you need a little more steam to reach your goals, or is there some fog that is hampering your progress? Does your life seem too dry or too humid or too damp?

The **Odor** metaphor for the Earth Element is **Fragrant**. We might think of taking time to smell the flowers, to appreciate the pleasant and enjoyable aspects of life. One traditional association with the Fragrant metaphor is the smell of incense in spiritual or cultural celebrations. We might think of the smells we associate with our own family or cultural holidays.

What does Fragrant symbolize in your life? Are you taking enough time to "stop and smell the flowers"-- appreciate the Fragrance in your life-- or do you need to focus on following through with your work, making the effort to bring in the harvest?

The **Taste** metaphor of the Earth Element is **Sweet.** This can be related to all the senses in addition to the sensation of pleasure in the mouth. Sweet can be a pleasing smell as with Fragrance, a sound that is melodious or harmonious to the ear as with Singing, a pleasing, beautiful, well-formed vision for the eye, or even a characteristic of being amiable, good-natured, gentle, welcome or Sympathetic. The metaphor of a Sweet Taste can symbolize many aspects of our life in addition to the literal sweet taste of foods and the possible dietary, social, cultural and other meanings tastes can have for us.

What tastes Sweet in your life, or in relation to your goals? Do need to have more, or just appreciate more, the sweet aspects of your life in order to achieve your goals?

Earth Element Metaphors

The **Emotion** metaphor of the Earth Element is **Sympathy** or Empathy. This is the emotion of compassion that involves sharing of feelings with another and/or understanding another's feelings or experience and responding appropriately. This can be an expression of condolence and comforting in times of grief or sadness, but it can also be a spirit of kinship, camaraderie, or like-mindedness in relation to any emotion. In balance, Sympathy or Empathy allow us to understand where others are "coming from". Out of balance, we can be overwhelmed by the attitudes and emotions of others and lose our own emotional balance.

How might Sympathy/Empathy relate to your goals? Are you being too sympathetic or empathetic and losing sight of your own feelings and needs, or do you need to relate more to the feelings of other? Do you need more/less empathy/sympathy from others?

The **Sound** metaphor of the Earth Element is **Singing**. The metaphor of singing involves uttering and/or hearing of words with rhythmic or musical modulation of the voice. As with the metaphor of Empathy, it can express, relate to, or inspire any of the Emotions. The idea of singing can simply mean uttering an expressive sound. Singing relates to self-expression and understanding of others. We all have moments when we need sing, to proclaim our own feelings, or feel the need for enthusiastic praise from others. A person with a recurring imbalance of the Singing aspect of the Earth Element often says, "I can't sing" or, "I never sing." This may relate literally to (hidden) wounds related to singing ability, or it may relate to our ability to express ourselves, to be understood, or to understand others.

What does Singing mean to you in your life, or in relation to your goal? Do you feel like you "sing" or tell too much, or do you need more enthusiastic, expressive singing in your life?

The Earth Element is said to **Fortify the Muscles**. The Muscles symbolize movement and activity. To Fortify the Muscles might make you stronger, more developed, or more powerful? More agile, more flexible, or more active?

What role does Muscle or strength play in your goals? Do you need more power, movement or activity to reach your goals or do you need to focus more on centeredness, stillness and patience?

The **Personal Power** metaphor of the Earth Element is **Decrease**. There is a point in our lives when less is more and we need to let go of some things to have more power in our own life. There are many aspects of cutting back or gradual diminution in our lives that allow us to be more effective and more authentic.

What in your life is no longer necessary, fruitful or beneficial that you continue to keep or do out of habit or fear of change? What can you let go of that would allow you to have more Personal Power in your life?

The **Faith/Worldview** metaphor of the Earth Element relates to Late Adolescence and Early Adulthood. Structure and function are seen in context. Systems are seen to reflect flexible and multiple purposes. This is a transitional phase characterized by disillusionment with literalism and blind acceptance of rules. Instead we increase our abilities of abstract thinking and reflection upon the self and one's own actions from multiple/others' perspectives. It can be called the **Conventional/Synthetic Faith** Worldview.

Are you placing too little or too much reliance on the values of your peer group, community or culture and seeing yourself through the eyes of others? Are you bogged down and stuck in your own thoughts and feelings, or are you in denial of your true inner thoughts and feelings about your experience of life?

STOMACH: 7-9 AM

Neck Flexors & Extensors: Niacin, B6, G, Iodine
Pectoralis Major Clavicular: B, G, HCl
Levator Scapulae: B
Brachioradialis: B

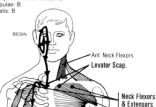

BEGIN

Ant. Neck Flexors
Levator Scap.

Neck Flexors & Extensors
Pect. Maj. Clav.

5-6
**Pect. Maj. Clav.
Brachioradialis**
Left side only

Brachioradialis

39   C-5 or T-8

Levator Scapulae

43

Brachioradialis

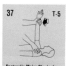

37   T-5

Pectoralis Major Clavicular
(Sitting, Laying or Standing)

41   C-2

Ant. Neck Flexors (Sinuses)

41

Ant. Neck Flexors (Sinuses)

41

Post. Neck Ext. (Sinuses)

41

Post. Neck Ext. (Sinuses)

C-2

C7-T1
Lev.
Scapulae

Neck Flexors & Ext.
Neck Extensors

5-6

**Pect. Maj.
Clavicular**

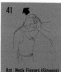

To Strengthen

FIRST
S 41   SI 5
S 43
GB 41
SECOND

To Weaken

SECOND
FIRST
S 43
GB 41   LI 1
S 45

Stomach Meridian Function 7-9 AM

The Stomach Function involves receiving potential nutrients and beginning the digestive functions. The 35 million cells in the stomach have multiple functions. The Stomach Function is taking in new materials and new ideas, mixing them and temporarily storing them for further assimilation. It is a moment in the cycle of seeing what is available and tagging it for use in other functions of the Soul. The Stomach Meridian is particularly associated with the mouth as the beginning of the digestive system, but must necessarily involve the sense of smell, vision, etc. As it is often said, digestion truly begins in the brain and the Stomach Function has a strong mental/emotional component as well as a dietary component. We come into first contact with potential nutrients and new ideas through what we see, smell or hear and digestion occurs best when it involves a full appreciation with the five senses. Sometimes we don't see what we're taking in (watch what we eat), or we swallow something without chewing, or without realizing that it's poison. We may need to think more about what we're taking in, or even vomit it up, or at least allow ourselves the time to digest it, whether it's a food, a feeling, a thought, etc.

Are you receiving the proper resources to fulfill your purposes? Are you able to use your resources efficiently? What nutrient, emotion, or idea are you digesting? What is difficult for you to swallow or gives you a stomachache (physical, emotional, etc) or inhibits free breathing, figuratively or literally?

Muscles Associated with the Stomach Meridian

Muscle: PECTORALIS MAJOR CLAVICULAR—

This chest muscle helps bend and turn the arm at the shoulder. Contracting this muscle also elevates and opens the chest. This muscle is particularly associated with the Stomach Meridian Function (and emotional function) of processing and digesting incoming material. We prefer to start balancing with the Stomach meridian after the Central and Governing meridians because the

Stomach - PMC

emotional/digestive component is so frequently a crucial component in our goal-balancing process.

Feel this muscle contracting at the top of your chest between the shoulder and the area below the collarbone.

Test: Position the straight arm 90° from the body, palm out and thumb toward the feet. Pressure is on the forearm to bring the arm 45° down and out from the body.

In relation to your goal, do you need to hold your chest up and be more proud or are you too proud?

Muscle: LEVATOR SCAPULAE-
This muscle has its origin in the first four cervical vertebrae. It has a major role in keeping the head held up and even. Inhibition in these muscles can result in the head dropping forward, and or twisting or tilting to one side.

Feel this muscle contracting between your mid neck and the inner/medial top of the shoulder blade, deep in that area.

Test: With the elbow bent and forced down against the side of the hip, pressure is against the inside of the upper arm near the elbow to pull the arm away from the side.

Are you having difficulty keeping your head on straight literally or figuratively? Would you say that you have your nose too high in the air or don't seem to be able to hold your head high?

Muscle: NECK MUSCLES-
NOTE: There are so many muscles involved in the neck that it is a very subtle practice trying to isolate, sense and test any individual muscle. This parallels the relation of the neck muscles to the stomach meridian, which is associated with emotions. The neck muscles are all

involved in the subtle changes in facial expressions involved in emotions. Pay attention to the facial expressions when testing the neck muscles and see what metaphors are generated.

(Anterior Neck flexors)-
These muscles are found in the front and sides of the neck. They help to hold the head up and keep the ears and shoulders level. They are particularly vulnerable to injury from whiplash. They are also related to the functioning of the sinuses, which are important in drainage from the head and scalp as well as immune responses.

Feel these muscles contracting in the front and anterior sides of your neck as you bring your head forward.

Test: Bring the head forward, bracing between the shoulder blades if standing. Pressure is against the forehead to extend the head. Check also with flexed head turned 10° and 45° to each side, exerting pressure each time at the highest point of the forehead.

Note: If the person is uncomfortable about having their neck muscles tested, do not test, but show them the correction reflexes and notice if moving the head through the range of motion is more comfortable after working the reflexes.

Are you having trouble holding your head up, literally or figuratively? Are you looking at things evenly, or are you tilted to one side? Have you suffered any literal or figurative whiplash? How is the air effecting you? Is it literally or figuratively stale, fresh, stinky, or fragrant? Is your head (life) clogged, literally or figuratively, or are you feeling a steady flow of fresh air to clear your head?

(Posterior Neck Extensors)-
These muscles are found in the back and sides of the neck. They help to hold the head back over the shoulders. If they are inhibited, the head tends to pull forward like a turtle sticking its head out.

Feel these muscles contracting at the back of your neck and the posterior sides of your neck as your bring your head back.

Test: Bring the head back, bracing at the top of the chest if standing. Pressure is against the back of the head to push it forward. Check also with head turned to each side.

Note: If the person is uncomfortable about having their neck muscles tested, do not test, but show them the correction reflexes and notice if moving the head through the range of motion is more comfortable after working the reflexes.

Observe your posture. Are you literally sticking your neck out? Figuratively, are you taking too many risks, or do you need to take more chances?

Muscle: BRACHIORADIALIS-
This muscle flexes the elbow and helps turn the wrist. If it is inhibited, it may be difficult to get the arm up and behind the back.

Feel this small muscle contracting between your arm and forearm at the Elbow when the thumb is pointed to the shoulder.

Test: Arm is bent to slightly more than 90°, thumb toward shoulder. Brace at the elbow. Pressure is on the thumb side of the wrist to straighten the arm.

Are you able to reach behind you to get important things done? Can you scratch your own back or are there areas where you're dependent on others? Do you feel like someone is twisting your arm back, or is there something going on behind your back that you can't "get hold of"? Are you flexible in your outlook, or only looking straight ahead, ignoring your blindspot?

Stomach - Brachioradialis

104

Testimonials

Touch for Health is a simple yet powerful system that anyone can learn to use to balance their own energy and help others

My family has adopted Dr. Thie's vision to use this method of balancing the body daily. After taking the TFH Intensive seminar, my husband and I have benefited more that we could ever explain to anyone, emotionally, physically and spiritually.
—Teri Dauk

The holistic approach of TFH is amazing and yet very simple. The ability to treat an individual as a whole unit (mind, body and spirit) is the most innovative approach towards personal health that I've ever seen. I would strongly recommend TFH for anyone interested in improving or maintaining their own personal wellness.
—Paul Farinha

TFH works amazingly quietly to balance and center the body, emotions and spirit. Results can be seen and felt immediately. These powerful techniques can be learned by a layperson in a short period of time. As a professor, author and clairvoyant teacher I know little about physiology but was able to use TFH as soon as I completed the TFH Intensive seminar. I learned effective specific tools to assist myself and others to achieve balance.
—Gayle Kimball PhD

SPLEEN: 9-11 AM

Latissimus Dorsi: A, F, HCl
Triceps: A
Opponens Pollicis Longus: B6, A
Lower Trapezius: F, G, C
Trapezius: C

½" above post. fontanel

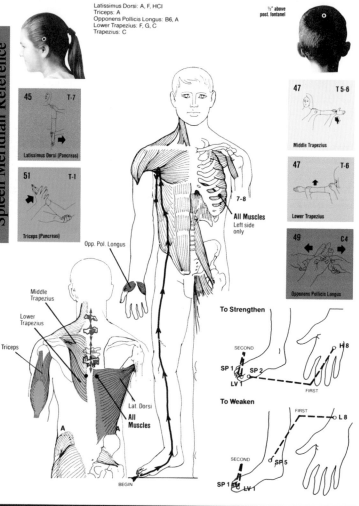

45 T-7
Latissimus Dorsi (Pancreas)

51 T-1
Triceps (Pancreas)

47 T 5-6
Middle Trapezius

47 T-6
Lower Trapezius

49 C4
Opponens Pollicis Longus

Opp. Pol. Longus

7-8

All Muscles
Left side only

Middle Trapezius
Lower Trapezius
Triceps

Lat. Dorsi
All Muscles

A A

BEGIN

To Strengthen

SECOND
SP 1 SP 2
LV 1
FIRST
H 8

To Weaken

FIRST
L 8
SECOND
SP 5
SP 1 LV 1

Spleen Meridian Function 9-11 AM

While the stomach receives raw materials, the spleen functions to transform them into useable forms and to distribute them. It is a moment in the cycle of assimilating what is appropriate and identifying toxic or harmful elements to be eliminated. Spleen Function also relates to immune functions, purifying the blood, increasing power of the white blood cells and removing the damaged and dead red blood cells. Pancreas function is also related to the Spleen Meridian and is involved in sugar metabolism, particularly, and digestion in general, breaking things down into manageable parts.

Are you burdening yourself with toxic materials and overworking the detox/immune system function in dietary, mental, chemical or spiritual areas? Do you have enough sweetness or too much sweetness? How are you at breaking down problems into digestible parts?

Muscles Associated with the Spleen Meridian

Muscle: LATISSIMUS DORSI-

This muscle extends from the hip to the spine and to the shoulder and is involved in all the movements of the arm across the front of the body. When it is out of balance posture is effected from the shoulders to the pelvis. This muscle is particularly associated with Pancreas function, having to do with sugar metabolism and digestion in general. The digestion metaphor has to do with breaking things down into manageable parts.

Feel this muscle contracting at the side of the back when the elbow is held tightly against the body, arm straight, with the thumb pointing to the back.

Spleen - Lat. Dorsi

Test: Position the straight arm beside the body, elbow in, palm out, thumb pointing back. Be sure there is no tension in the shoulder girdle. Pressure is at the forearm to pull the arm slightly forward and away from the body.

Are you taking swings, or striking at things, physically, mentally, emotionally and/or spiritually? Or are you inhibited from making large gestures in trying to reach your goals? Are you taking in too much sweet stuff, or not enough, literally or figuratively? How are you at breaking down problems into bite size chunks?

Muscle: MIDDLE TRAPEZIUS-

This is one of the muscles that keeps the shoulder blade in and turns it. The motion of the test suggests opening your arms as wide as possible to take in or embrace as much as possible. This muscle is particularly associated with Spleen Meridian Function, which relates to immune functions and cleaning up the blood increasing power of the white blood cells function and removing the damaged and old red blood cells.

Feel this muscle contracting between the posterior part of the shoulder and the spine from the middle of the spine to the neck with your arms fully extended at shoulder level and brought back toward the spine, palms facing forwards.

Test: Hold the arm straight out to the side and the thumb toward the head. Pressure is against the back of the wrist to push it forwards while holding the shoulder down.

Are you attempting to embrace too much, or do you need to open your arms wide to embrace all of your life? How are you doing with keeping your act cleaned up?

Muscle: LOWER TRAPEZIUS—

This is one of the muscles that keeps the shoulder blade in and turns it. The motion of the test suggests opening your arms above you to grasp or hold up something above you. This muscle is particularly associated with Spleen Meridian Function, which relates to immune functions and cleaning up the blood increasing power of the white blood cells function and removing the damaged and old red blood cells. How are you doing with keeping your act cleaned up?

Feel this muscle contracting between the posterior part of the shoulder and the spine from the middle of the spine to area where the low back curve begins with your arms fully extended and brought back toward the spine and slightly towards your feet, palms facing the head.

Test: Hold the arm straight out to the side and the palm facing toward the head. Pressure is at the wrist to press the arm headward.

Are you attempting to grasp or hold up too much, or do you need to open your arms wide to embrace the whole sky? Are you burdening yourself with toxic materials and overworking the Spleen/detox/immune system function in dietary, mental, chemical or spiritual areas?

Muscle: OPPONENS POLLICIS LONGUS-

This test gives us an indication of the relative function of the grip of the opposing little finger and thumb. This muscle is particularly associated with Pancreas function, having to do with sugar metabolism and digestion functions of breaking things down into manageable parts, and separating what is useful and what is not.

Feel this muscle contracting at the palm side of the thumb when holding the little finger and thumb together.

Test: Hold the tip of the thumb to tip of little finger, making a ring. Test by pulling thumb and little finger apart. A little bit of separation on the test is normal; check to see if the muscles lock after coming apart just a bit. If so, the muscle may be considered strong.

What do you need to get a grip on? What are you holding on to too tightly or not tightly enough? What are you hanging on to that you need to let go of? Are you taking in too much sweet stuff, or not enough, literally or figuratively? How are you at breaking down problems into bite size chunks?

Muscle: TRICEPS-

This muscle at the back of the arm helps to straighten the arm, working opposite the biceps.

The motion of the test suggests reaching out or drawing in. This muscle is particularly associated with Pancreas function, having to do with sugar metabolism and digestion in general. The digestion metaphor has to do with breaking things down into manageable parts.

Feel this muscle contracting on the posterior of the arm between the elbow and the shoulder when you extend your forearm straightening it out at the elbow, hand facing the body.

Test with the arm partly flexed. Brace the elbow. Pressure is against the back of the wrist to bend it further. ON children, start with the arm almost straight.

Are you reaching out enough or not enough, literally or figuratively? Are you gathering in too much or too little? Are you taking in too much sweet stuff, or not enough, literally or figuratively? How are you at breaking down problems into bite size chunks?

The Fire Element
Heart, Small Intestine, Circulation-Sex and Triple Warmer

The **Fire Element** can be represented by the image of the hot, red sun, giving both light and warmth. It is associated with all of life's heat and passions, particularly with enthusiasm, vitality and "warm feelings". The Wood element provides the fuel for Fire and the Earth Element is formed from the ashes generated by Fire. Fire controls the Metal Element by melting it, purifying it, or forging it and giving it shape and strength. Water controls Fire by tempering or quenching it.

When you think of Fire, what image comes to mind and what might this symbolize in your life? Do you have enough "fire in the belly", passion and energy for life? Are you too passionate, burning up your energy stores, burning those around you, or are you too cold, and unable to be passionate?

The Color metaphor associated with the Fire Element is Red. This is the red of fire, of burning passions, of fuels converted into energy.

What does the color Red mean to you in your life, related to your current life goals? Do you have enough Red in your life, or too much Red?

The **Season** metaphor of the Fire Element is **Summer**. Summer is the warmest season and is the time of the most daylight. It is expected to be the period of finest development or maturing of powers. It can relate to the time for vacations and having fun or the early harvesting of the fast maturing crops. Perhaps greater activity is resulting in more vitality, fitness, muscle strength and tone.

What does the Summer mean in your life? What could Summer symbolize in relation to your goal? Are you able to have "fun in the sun", enjoying the warmth and activity of Summer, or are you

sensitive to light, sapped of energy? Could you be exerting too much energy, getting burned by the light and heat of sun?

The **Climate** metaphor for the Fire Element is **Heat**. Imagine a place or a time when the dominant climate is heat. We can think of the heat of the Summer, or heat may relate to great passions, high pressure, or danger. When it's very hot, we need to balance the heat by drinking plenty of water, and so we must balance the Fire Element with the Water Element.

What might Heat symbolize in your life? Can you withstand the Heat in your job, family life, community etc. or is the stress and pressure overwhelming? Do you adapt to pressure and crises with adequate counterbalancing measures? Are you too passionate, playing it too cool, or getting burned out?

The **Odor** associated with the Fire Element is **Scorched**. The Scorched smell can be associated with a superficial burn or shriveling. This might mean a literal scorching by the hot sun, or any harsh weather, or a metaphorical "trial by fire", taking risks and surviving dangerous situations with minimal consequences. Scorched might also relate to severe criticism, scorn, or stigma.

What does a Scorched smell suggest to you? Have you been literally scorched by fire or the elements, or scorched by traumatic experiences, or the passions, demands, or criticisms of others? Do you need to take some risky actions, even at the cost of getting a little scorched?

The **Taste** associated with the Fire Element is **Bitter**. Bitter is the taste of many poisons and may indicate danger. Many natural stimulants have a Bitter flavor. We use bitter as a metaphor for lingering regrets or a sense of injustice or unpleasantness.

What does a Bitter taste make you think of? Do you have a

lingering regret or grudge that you're Bitter about? What's poisoning you, or adding a bitter element to your pleasures? Are you over-stimulated, on edge, hooked on adrenaline, ready to fight or flee at any moment, or do you need some stimulation in your life to get the juices flowing?

The **Emotion** associated with the Fire Element is **Joy**. Joy may be a keen and lively pleasure, getting a kick out of life, or satisfaction with your life and having a sense of peace and well being. The Fire element is also associated with all of the passionate emotions, particularly Love. It's important to be aware when we are lacking happiness, feeling spiritless, gloomy, or downhearted. There are four meridians associated with the Fire element but only two associated with the other elements. From this we might infer that, although it's important to allow ourselves to experience all of the emotions, we need to have at least twice as much Love and Joy as the other emotions. However, when we are manic or jovial when it's not appropriate, oblivious to circumstances that require a shift in attitude other than "happy-go-lucky", it can be a problem.

What place does Joy have in your life and how does Joy relate to your goals? Do you need more Love and Joy in your life, or are you masking pain with a manic attitude that is out of touch with reality? Are you dependent on drugs, etc. to stimulate you and allow you to enjoy yourself, or can you find contentment within yourself?

The **Sound** associated with the Fire Element is **Laughing**. This sound is made by rhythmically exhaling in a spirit of mirth, joy, or pleasure. Laughter can also be associated with triumph, ridicule, or defiance etc. Laughter can be one of the most healing forms of expression, but we may need to unlearn negative associations with laughter , such as "laughing is for fools" or traumatic experiences where we have been the object of derisive laughter. Laughter may also come at strange moments, when we are nervous, frightened, grieving or in despair.

Paying attention to the spirit behind the laughter can be very important for our healing.

What role does Laughing have in your life or in relation to your goal? Do you need to have more mirth and Laughing in your life, or do you avoid experiencing other emotions by "laughing them off"? Is there something that you need to allow yourself to laugh about, or have you laughed at an inappropriate moment? Have you been made fun of, laughed at, scorned or ridiculed?

The Fire Element is said to **Fortify the Arteries**. The Arteries circulate our lifeblood, bringing nourishment and fuel. This might literally relate to circulation, immune system function, and the maintenance of body temperature. It can relate figuratively to our supply lines of essential materials, fuel for heat and cooking, food supplies and anything that sustains our life.

What do Arteries or Supply Lines symbolize in relation to your goals? Do you have a steady flow of the fuels and supplies that you need to maintain your mental, emotional, spiritual and physical vitality? Are you able to distribute your resources to sustain all of the areas of your life, or do some parts of your life get poor circulation and go cold?

The **Personal Power** metaphor of the Fire Element is **Mature**. To mature is to reach your full growth, to come of age, to be able to use discretion. Maturity is characterized by a full appreciation and use of our capacities and an understanding of our limitations. To be fully mature is to be able to act responsibly without always worrying about whether our behavior seems "grown up". If we are precocious, we may have the appearance of being mature without the capacity to be responsible, or we may have knowledge and experience that is beyond our maturity.

What does Mature symbolize in your life, or in relation to your goals? Are you at ease with your limitations and able to make full use of your capacities? Are you being overly capricious or are you always acting "like and adult", and never experiencing the childlike wonder and joy in life?

In the **Faith/Worldview** metaphor of the Fire Element is related to Childhood or "School Years". This phase is characterized by the **Mechanistic, Circular Causality** model where linear thinking sees all effects as directly related to causes that precede them. This is the belief that, "If you just look carefully enough, you will find the single cause for any given effect." One will find the specific germ, virus or gene that is causing the specific effect (disease as a discrete entity that can be killed). It is a warrior model where there are good guys and bad guys and fighting is the best way to reach your goal. It is referred to as the **Literal/Mythic** stage. In this stage we are given to literal interpretation of moral rules and attitudes and favor a singularity of meaning, in which fact is distinguished from and valued over fantasy. There is a focus on Reciprocity and a tendency to Perfectionism.

What does Literal or Mythic Faith suggest to you? Are you hemmed in by a narrow, literal interpretation of rules, morals or beliefs or could you benefit from being conscious of conventions and not always having to re-invent the wheel or go it alone? Do you expect precise reciprocity in your dealings with others?

PLEASE NOTE: The Circulation Sex and Triple Warmer Meridians are also related to the Fire element, but follow the Kidney Meridian in the 24-Hour Cycle. Refer back to the above Fire element metaphors for these meridians, as well as Heart and Small Intestine.

Fire Element Metaphors

Heart Meridian Reference

HEART: 11 AM-1 PM

G, E, B, Calcium

53   T-2

Subscapularis

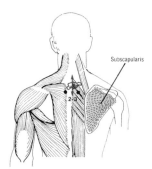

Subscapularis

2-3

To Strengthen

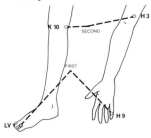

K 10 ○ - - - SECOND - - - ○ H 3

FIRST

LV ○

H 9

To Strengthen Small Intestine Meridian in lieu of weakening heart

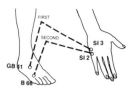

FIRST

SECOND

SI 3

SI 2

GB 41

B 66

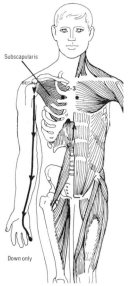

Subscapularis

BEGIN   2-3

Down only

Heart Meridian Function 11 AM-1 PM

The Heart Function involves the cycling of the blood as well as electrical communication with the rest of the cells of the whole Soul. The heart is in constant communication with all of the organs and muscles to determine their blood/oxygen needs from moment to moment. The heart generates 5000 times more powerful electrical messages throughout the Soul than the brain. In the Chinese belief system, the heart is also strongly associated with mental processes, while in the West we have the traditional metaphor of the heart as an emotional center and a center of wisdom. In Chinese medicine, the heart is called the "sovereign ruler" which directs action with clear insight.

How is your circulation and communication within your Soul, or in your daily activities, literally or figuratively? What do you feel in your heart as opposed to your head? Is there any conflict between your logical thinking, intuition, wisdom or emotional feelings? How are you functioning in relation to receiving and sending messages about your life to yourself and others?

Muscle Associated with the Heart Meridian

SUBSCAPULARIS-

This muscle functions to hold the shoulder blade in place. It is hidden behind the shoulder blade, and so cannot be observed or felt by another person, accept by secondary inference. This muscle is particularly associated with Heart Meridian Function, which involves the circulation of the blood and electrical communication throughout the whole Soul, as well as the traditional metaphor of the heart as an emotional center.

Heart - Subscapularis

Feel this muscle contracting under the shoulder blade when the arm is held at ninety degrees from the side of the body and the forearm is held to form a right angle and pulled posterior to feel the contraction of the muscle. It can also be felt by placing the back of the hand at the small of the back and pressing it against the body and feeling the contraction under the shoulder blade.

Test: Hold arm out to the side, with elbow bent to 90° and level with the shoulder, hand toward the feet. Brace at the elbow to stabilize the arm. Pressure is at the forearm to bring the forearm up towards the head.

What are you hiding or keeping private? Is there something that you need to reveal? What do you feel in your heart as opposed to your head? How are you in receiving and sending messages about your life to yourself and others? How is your communication and circulation within your Soul, or in your daily activities, literally or figuratively?

Heart - Subscapularis

Testimonials
Touch for Health is a powerful tool for all kinds of health practitioners

As a certified kinesiologist, a massage therapist and a personal trainer, I find TFH extremely helpful. It gives me a whole new way of looking at my clients and my profession and a new excitement for helping others. Experiencing Dr. Thie's class has definitely made me a more confident and knowledgeable practitioner. I would recommend TFH for anyone who is interested in helping others to achieve their physical, emotional, mental or spiritual goals. I got several wonderful balances that helped to clear issues that I was not even aware that I was hanging on to.
>   —Kaayla Cevan Braverman

TFH has helped me on many levels to accept and cherish myself. In a very real way I feel that it is helping me to grow up and take responsibility for myself, for my health and for my physical comfort. I have often felt overwhelmed by goal setting in the past and TFH has shown me how important and easy it is to set a realistic and personal goal which can easily become integrated in my life by applying the TFH methods. Dr. Thie is truly a master and has modeled how to become more congruent, honest, loving, accepting, compassionate, confident and joyful in my life!! I feel confident that I will apply TFH in my life and in my work. Blessings to you and many, many thanks.
>   —Robert Bearden RN

TFH is great for self healing as well as learning the techniques to balance muscles by setting goals to release emotional, mental, physical and spiritual stress in the body (and then using the techniques to balance).
>   —Marge Jones, ND

SMALL INTESTINE: 1-3 PM

Abdominals: E
Quadriceps: D, B

Pull apart for Rectus
and Transverse Abdominis

8-9
9-10
10-11

L-5

BEGIN

Quadriceps
Rect. Abdominis
Trans. Abdominis

Transverse
Both sides

Quadriceps

Rectus
Both sides

57   T-6
Rectus Abdominis

57
Rectus Abdominis

57   T-6
Transverse Abdominis

57
Transverse Abdominis

To Weaken

To Strengthen

FIRST
SI 3
SI 2
GB 41
B 66   SECOND

S 36   SI 8
FIRST
SECOND
B 66   SI 2

55
Quadriceps

55   T-10
Quadriceps

Small Intestine Meridian Function 1-3 PM

The Small Intestine Function is primarily absorption of nutritious substances and the separation of waste material. These same functions take place on the cellular level, and in the Soul as a whole. It is the assimilation of influences and stuff from outside the Soul. The small intestine winds for over 23 feet and has three main parts, the duodenum, the jejunum, and the ileum. Throughout the small intestine, various secretions from other organs are added to the liquefied foods, which aid in the absorption nutrients. Bacteria make up a large amount of the contents of the small intestine, also acting upon the materials that enter so that they can be absorbed.

Are you having trouble digesting or absorbing things in your life that are meant to be nourishing, literally or figuratively? What is difficult for you to absorb or gives you a stomachache (physical, emotional, etc) or inhibits free breathing, figuratively or literally?

Muscles Associated with the Small Intestine Meridian

Muscle: QUADRICEPS-

This muscle straightens the knee and flexes the thigh. Weakness will be evident when there is difficulty climbing stairs or getting up from a seated position. Pain in the knee is often associated with weakness in this muscle. This muscle is also associated with the function of the jejunum and ileum, which are the last 2/3 of the small intestine, and weakness in this muscle may correspond with digestive problems.

Feel this muscle in the front of your thigh when you bend your thigh at the hip as you would in taking a step up and keeping your foot in front, ahead of your knee.

Test: Hold the thigh not quite at 90° to the body, knee bent with foot in front of the knee. Pressure is at the knee and the ankle to push the leg downward to straighten it. Do not allow the thigh to twist, substituting Fascia Lata.

What do you need to step up to or are you taking steps that are too large? What in your life is like climbing stairs or climbing a mountain? Are you having trouble digesting or absorbing things in your life that are meant to be nourishing, literally or figuratively?

Muscle: ABDOMINALS-

These muscles are associated with posture and are very important in maintaining a balanced spine. When these muscles are out of balance, many pains in the back and neck can be present. They are always used together and are thin layers that allow for twisting and bending and maintaining the abdominal contents in the best positions for full functioning. These muscles need exercise. One of the best exercises for them is walking with a long stride. Recovery from the postural changes during pregnancy will be enhanced by strengthening these muscles and maintaining an exercise routine of at least 20 minutes daily which involve using these muscles. These muscles are also associated with the duodenum, the first third of the small intestine. They are commonly weak in connection with "stomach aches", digestion problems, and breathing difficulty.

Feel these muscles between your lowest ribs, breastbone and the pubic bone while seated with your feet as close to the buttocks as comfortable and leaning back with the chin level. The oblique and transverse can be felt best when twisting from this position to the left and right.

Rectus Abdominis Test: Sit with knees bent and together, hands on the opposite shoulders, leaning back, chin up. Pressure is against the wrists where they cross, to push backwards, Stabilize the thighs by placing a forearm above the knees as you test.

Standing: place hands on opposite shoulders. Ask the person to lean forward ensuring they do not flex their neck muscles. Brace firmly at the lower back. Pressure is against the arms at the midline to push straight back.

Transverse & Oblique Test: Sitting with knees bent, heels towards buttocks, arms crossed to opposite shoulders and torso twisted about 25° and leaning back, chin up. Brace on knees. Pressure is in two directions: first, to untwist the torso, and second, to push diagonally through from lower shoulder. When standing, person leans forward and twists torso about 25°, chin neutral, arms across shoulders. Tester braces firmly across lower back. First push to untwist the torso, then push through the angle of the shoulders.

What are you doing that is not allowing you to maintain the posture that is most suitable for you literally or figuratively? How is your attitude toward life in general, balanced or unbalanced? Do you feel that you are fulfilling your daily walk of life? What is difficult for you to absorb, gives you a stomachache (physical, emotional, etc) or inhibits free breathing, figuratively or literally?

Small Intestine- Abdominals

The Water Element
Bladder and Kidney Meridians

The **Water Element** is symbolized by the water of the oceans, seas, lakes, and rivers. The Metal Element is said to create water, which we might visualize as water condensing on a cold metal surface, or bubbling up from the same depths in the earth where ores and salts are condensed. Water is controlled by the Earth, which contains it and gives it form, and water controls fire by quenching it. Water is very mysterious and can take many forms. It is a symbol of the unconscious, of our dreamlife, of our emotions, of that which we do not understand and that which we fear. But it is also essential to our daily living and smooth functioning.

What does Water symbolize for you in your life or in the context of your goals? Is there too much mystery, fear and risk, or do you need to overcome your fears and allow some uncertainty to fulfill your dreams?

The Color associated with the Water Element is Blue. We might think of a blue color in water.

What does the color blue mean to you in your life or in relation to your current goals?

The **Season** associated with the Water Element is **Winter**. We might visualize a time of hibernation or a time of bleakness. It can be seen as a time of reintegration and repair and preparation for the coming time of planting and new beginnings. It is a time of decreased activity and greater attention to rest and internal reflection.

What does Winter mean in your life or related to your goals? Are you too active when you need to concentrate on quiet contemplation or planning? Do you feel left out in the cold, or do you have a warm place where you are safe and nurtured?

Water Element Metaphors

The **Climate** metaphor for the Water Element is **Cold**. We might picture the cold weather of winter, or a person who is "cold", apathetic, unemotional, lacking personal warmth.

What does Cold symbolize in your life or in relation to your goal? Are you numbed by a harsh environment, or do you need to cool your passions and be calm to achieve your objectives?

The **Odor** metaphor for the Water Element is **Putrid**. Imagine decaying flesh, which has a very foul, strong odor. Perhaps there is something in your life that has died and needs to be laid to rest. Or perhaps there is some decay or corruption in your life that is intolerable or may be fatal.

What does a Putrid or Stagnant smell signify in your life, or in relation to your goal? What has died and needs to be buried? What is thoroughly corrupt, offensively or disgustingly objectionable?

The **Taste** metaphor of the Water Element is **Salty**. The salinity of our blood plasma is almost precisely that of seawater, yet we cannot drink seawater and we must be careful about our salt intake. Salt is used to enhance the flavor of things, and also as a preservative, preventing meat, in particular, from becoming spoiled. We sometimes say, "take this with a grain of salt" when some information in not completely reliable.

What does a Salty Taste mean in your life and in relation to your goal? What needs to be preserved in your life, materially, spiritually, intellectually? What "needs some salt" or must be "taken with a grain of salt"?

The **Emotion** associated with the Water Element is **Fear**, Anxiety or Awe. We might picture the vast, unknown depths of the sea, or the deep fears within our subconscious and dreams.

Water Element Metaphors

What Fears do you have related to your goals in life? Is there too much mystery, fear and risk, or do you need to overcome your fears and allow some uncertainty to fulfill your dreams? Can you convert fear into awe and excitement related to risks and potentially great outcomes? Are you worrying too much, or do you need to pay attention to the dangers in your life?

The **Sound** metaphor of the Water Element is **Groaning**. Imagine a deep, inarticulate, sound expressing fear, pain, sympathy, anger, reluctance, or even joy or pleasure. Groaning can include deep sighs, moaning, grumbling, whining, etc.

What do you need to Groan about, or are you groaning, or complaining too much? What kind of Groaning would correspond to how you feel about your life? How are you Groaning as you work towards your goal? How will you Groan when you reach your goal?

The Water Element is said to **Fortify the Bones**. The bones create a structure that allows the muscles to move us in a highly controlled way. The bones also serve to protect some of our vital organs such as the brain, heart and lungs. The bones function as a hydraulic system that gains strength when the pressure is greatest and becomes more flexible as the pressure is released. When we have deep emotions, or strong intuition, we sometimes say that we "feel it in the bones." The bones are the slowest to decay, and often remain long after something has died.

What do your Bones tell you about your life and your current goals? Can you be rigid when you need to be, and flexible when it's appropriate? Do you have any "skeletons in your closet"?

The **Personal Power** Metaphor of the Water element is Emphasize. Imagine having reduced your efforts and activities to an optimum functional level. Now think of placing your main **emphasis** on a particular aspect of your life that best expresses who you are and what your purpose is.

What particular aspect of your life do you need to emphasize to reach your goal? Where are you putting too much emphasis so that it interferes with your energy flow? Is there something that you know will help you achieve your purpose that is being neglected?

The **Faith/World View** metaphor of the Water Element is related to Late Maturity and Death. It is characterized by a worldview of **Integrative Diversity** and involves the final integration into our life of a goal achieved, and the relinquishing of the old life that has been changed by changed circumstances. This is the phase of **Re-integrative Universalizing Faith**. In this phase, we rehabilitate all of the aspects of ourselves that have been left undeveloped, ignored, evaded, or denied. Paradoxes and Polar opposites are not seen as puzzles to be solved, but mysteries to be accepted and appreciated. Humans are seen as BOTH good and evil, shaped by circumstances AND personally responsible for their choices. God is personal and abstract. We sense a transcendent value of faith and community among all humanity and tend to sacrifice the personal, individual life for the benefit of all. This sense is extended in the "universalizing" stage to a fellowship among all beings and a connection with the ultimate environment.

How does your sense of the Universal relate to your life and to your present goals? Is this a time for you to let go of concern for personal success, failure, contradiction, or injustice and simply concentrate on the greater good, or do you need be proactive in your own interests?

Water Element Metaphors

128

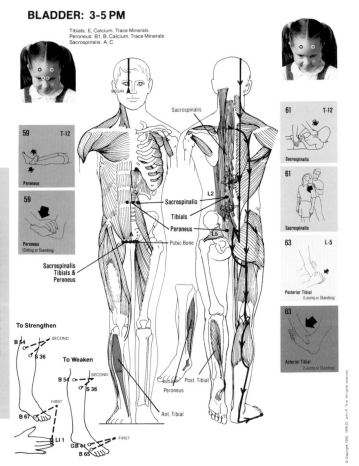

Bladder Reference

BLADDER: 3-5 PM

Tibials: E, Calcium, Trace Minerals
Peroneus: B1, B, Calcium, Trace Minerals
Sacrospinalis: A, C

BLADDER
6

Bladder Meridian Function 3-5 PM

The Bladder Function is to store waste liquid before elimination, not only in the urinary bladder but also in all of the cells and throughout the Soul. In the Chinese system, the Bladder is said to be the storehouse of emotions, and so the Bladder Function is involved in the water balance/emotional balance in the whole Soul. Water is eliminated as it reaches excessive volume, or when waste material is highly concentrated.

The urinary bladder is always "full" since the muscles expand or contract as more liquid is received from the kidneys. People often try to reduce the need to urinate by limiting their water intake, but are actually thwarted by the resulting concentration of the urine. By drinking more pure water, the bladder is actually strengthened through exercise of the expanding bladder muscles and there is actually LESS urgency to urinate since the waste materials are diluted. Water is a potent symbol for emotion and mystery in life, and the Bladder Function is also involved in the balance of mystery in the Soul. We sometimes try to eliminate mystery, ambiguity or emotion itself from our lives, only to become toxic in our certainties and rationalizations. When we are able to accept more of the vast mystery of existence, and allow our emotions to flow, we find our tolerance and flexibility are increased.

Although all of the Meridians have secondary pathways, the Bladder Meridian is the only one to have two main channels, and it is the longest Meridian, running in double channels along the full length of the spine.

Are you hydrated, lubricated and feeling a free flow of energy, or are you dry, tight, concentrated or inhibited? Are you able to stretch? What is an irritant, or is too highly concentrated and needs dilution and/or elimination? What emotion do you need to let flow? How are you coping with mystery, duality, paradox, or imperfections?

Bladder Meridian Metaphors

Muscles Associated with the Bladder Meridian

Muscle: PERONEUS

These muscles making up the Peroneal group are associated with the maintaining of foot and ankle balance. When they are inhibited, they can effect the entire posture by not allowing proper use of the foot, which results in an upward misuse, and misalignment of the entire posture.

Feel this group of muscles between the foot and the outer side of the calf when the little toe side of the foot is elevated as if trying to bring it toward the nose.

Test: Begin with toes turned to the side, little toe flexed toward the head. Ensure the big toe is not pulled up. Stabilize the foot by holding the heel in one hand. Pressure is against the outside of the foot just behind the toes, pressing down and in toward the midline while pushing up on the heel.

How are you mis-stepping literally or figuratively? Do you feel grounded and able to walk freely or do you need to watch your step? Are you using too much caution, pussyfooting around?

Muscle: SACROSPINALIS -

When these muscles are working in a balanced manner, you can lie on your belly and raise your entire chest off the ground in a posterior arch. This action helps the spinal discs get proper nourishment. These many small muscles work together to help keep the whole back erect. Weakness in these muscles is associated with 19 different areas of pain.

Feel these muscles, many small ones around the spine, when you lift your head backward and arch your entire spine to the back.

Bladder - Peroneus, Sacrospinalis

Test: Lying face down, both hands placed in the small of the back. Lift one shoulder, and look back over it. Pressure is against the back of the shoulder. Pressing it toward the table or floor while stabilizing the opposite hip. When standing, the person may be braced against a wall, or untwist at the shoulders.

What little things are causing you tension? What little things are keeping you from standing straight, literally or figuratively. Do you pay too much or too little attention to details?

Muscle: TIBIALS-

These muscles function to flex the foot out and upward. They are sometimes found inhibited when there are problems with the natural arches of the foot. These muscles are particularly associated with the urethra function of emptying the bladder and, in men, carrying the prostatic fluid/semen during ejaculation. The urethra is enwrapped by the prostate gland in men.

Anterior Tibial:

Feel this muscle on the outer side of the shinbone when you bring the big toe side of your foot toward your knee. Is it painful for you to release/let go of even toxic parts of your life? Do you have any issues around climaxing or orgasm, literally or figuratively?

Test: Hold the leg straight and the toes and ankle flexed toward the knee. Pressure is against the top of the foot to push the toes downward

Posterior Tibial:

This muscle is also sometimes associated with Triple Warmer Meridian and the adrenal function of "fight or flight" and the heat of passions.

Feel this muscle behind the shinbone when the foot is flexed away or down and inward.

Test: Hold the foot turned in and down as far as possible. Stabilize at the heel. Pressure is up and out on the ball of the foot just below the big toe.

How are you losing your balance? When you are thrown off balance do you recover quickly enough or not quickly enough for the situation or context? Are you kicking/being kicked, literally or figuratively? Is it painful for you to release/let go of even toxic parts of your life? Do you have any issues around climaxing or orgasm, literally or figuratively? Are you running or fighting to maintain your passion (for what)?

Bladder - Tibials

Testimonials
Touch for Health is helpful for psychotherapists, teachers, dancers & athletes

TFH is extremely useful both personally and professionally….I'm excited about integrating TFH in my psychotherapy practice.
—Karen Hansen

TFH is very valuable to me as a dancer, dance educator and personal trainer. I am now equipped with very practical knowledge and methods for helping my students, clients, colleagues and myself. TFH has brought me closer to my life goals with reassurance and calmness.
—Karen Scherwood

TFH has given me a greater understanding of muscles, the meridian system and muscle balancing. I will use this not only to improve my own performance as an athlete, but am excited to let my friends know of this technique and how it can help them.
—Alexis Waddel

I feel the metaphors will make a big impact on how I use TFH in the office. I think all CA's and CMT's should learn TFH so they can help the Dr. & patients in the office and at home.
—Paul McManus CMT

TFH is practical, reasonably easy to learn and highly effective. It offers a "big picture" approach to improving one's health. Holistic empowering "based on hope not disease." The training participants experience their own transformation from the process rather than just the "how to"(mechanics) .
—Marilyn Freeman HHP

KIDNEY: 5-7 PM

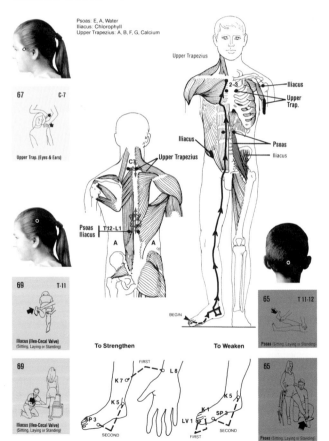

Psoas: E, A, Water
Iliacus: Chlorophyll
Upper Trapezius: A, B, F, G, Calcium

67   C-7

Upper Trap. (Eyes & Ears)

69   T-11

Iliacus (Ileo-Cecal Valve)
(Sitting, Laying or Standing)

69

Iliacus (Ileo-Cecal Valve)
(Sitting, Laying or Standing)

Upper Trapezius

C7

Upper Trapezius

Psoas
Iliacus   T12-L1

A   A

Upper Trapezius

Iliacus

Iliacus

Upper Trap.

Psoas

Iliacus

BEGIN

To Strengthen

FIRST

L 8

K 7

K 5

SP 3

SECOND

To Weaken

K 5

K 1

LV 1   SP 3

FIRST   SECOND

65   T 11-12

Psoas (Sitting, Laying or Standing)

65

Psoas (Sitting, Laying or Standing)

Kidney Reference

Kidney Meridian Function 5-7 PM

The Kidney Meridian Function is involved in controlling the volume, composition, and pressure of fluids in all the cells as well the whole Soul and is important in growth, development and reproductive functions. Blood flows through the kidneys at its highest pressure, toxins are filtered out, and nourishing materials are directed to where they are needed. Water is symbolic of mystery, emotion and spirit. Kidney Meridian Function is involved in the balance of these aspects of life. In Chinese medicine the Kidney is also said to be a storehouse of life force and has a strong spiritual aspect.

Where are you feeling pressure in your life, literally or figuratively? Are you bringing in enough fresh clear water to keep your life composition and volume in balance spiritually, emotionally, or physically? Do you feel that you have sufficient vitality for continued growth and development, or are you operating on reserve energy and just surviving?

Muscles Associated with the Kidney Meridian

Muscle: PSOAS-

This muscle both flexes the thigh on the trunk and the trunk on the thigh, thus it has paradoxical origins and insertions depending on the action in which it is used. This muscle is used both in sitting up motions and kicking to the side, or sidestepping motions. This muscle is particularly associated with the Kidney Meridian Function of maintaining the balance of the volume, composition, and pressure of fluids in each cell, as well as the body as a whole.

Feel this muscle contracting between the inside lateral portion of all the lumbar vertebrae and the inner portion of the upper thigh at the groin. The Quadriceps muscle is a synergistic muscle and if it is painful or felt strongly contracting in the test position use caution and consider this an indicator of an inhibition of the Psoas.

Kidney - Psoas

Test: Raise straight leg 45° up and to the side (or higher, if comfortable), and rotate laterally. Brace on the opposite hip. Pressure is against the inside of leg just above the ankle to push the leg back and out. If standing, use a wall or a chair to balance yourself.

What does the motion of kicking suggest to you, literally or figuratively? Is there any paradoxical aspect to your goal? Is there something you need to "sit up" and take notice of? In what aspect of your life do you feel the most pressure, literally or figuratively? Are you drinking enough water, or doing what you need to do for purification, spiritually, emotionally, mentally or physically?

Muscle: UPPER TRAPEZIUS-
This muscle tilts the chin and pulls in the shoulder blade. This muscle is also associated with symptoms related to the eyes and ears and when they are present the inhibition may be found with repeated muscle testing.

Feel this muscle contracting when tilting your head to the side with the nose pointing straightforward and raising your shoulder to the ear. It is a superficial muscle and quite strong.

Test: Tilt the head to the side (not turned) and the bring the shoulder up to meet the ear. Pressure is against the shoulder and the side of the head to pull them apart.

How do you feel that your head isn't on straight? Do you have difficulty "seeing straight" or keeping your head straight, literally or figuratively?

Muscle: ILIACUS-
The motion of this muscle test suggests kicking something aside. It is a small muscle that never the less may affect a wide range of movements. This muscle is also associated with the function of the transfer of nutrients and wastes from the small intestine to large

Kidney - Upper Trap.s, Iliacus

intestine at the cecum. When these functions are not normal it can result in symptoms almost anywhere. When vague symptoms are present this muscle may be an indicator of this energy imbalance in the subtle energy functions of the kidney meridian and its relationship to the large intestine meridian in all of the cells. This may be thought of as subtle energy imbalances in the process of eliminating waste material.

Feel this muscle inside the pelvis contracting at its attachment on the inside of the femur when the knee is bent at ninety degrees on the thigh and the foot and leg are turned to the side of the body as far as possible.

Test: Bend knee to 90 degrees, and turn lower leg as far out as to the side as possible. Pressure is at the ankle to bring leg toward the midline, while stabilizing the knee.

Is there something that needs to be kicked aside, or do you feel kicked aside? Are you throwing away things that are still useful, or are you hanging on to too much waste material, or do you have waste material in the wrong place, literally or figuratively? Is a subtle aspect of your life affecting various other parts of your life in unexpected ways?

Kidney - Iliacus

CIRCULATION-SEX: 7-9 PM

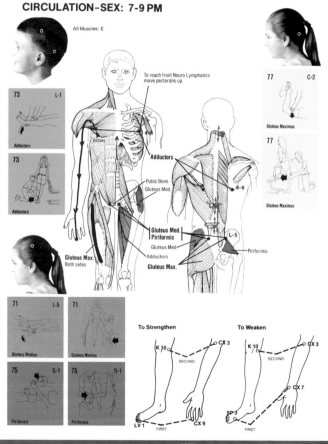

All Muscles: E

To reach front Neuro Lymphatics move pectoralis up.

73 L-1
Adductors

73
Adductors

77 C-2
Gluteus Maximus

77
Gluteus Maximus

Adductors

Pubic Bone
Gluteus Med.

Gluteus Med.
Piriformis
Gluteus Med
Adductors

Gluteus Max.
Both sides

Gluteus Max.

Piriformis

8-9

L-5

71 L-5
Gluteus Medius

71
Gluteus Medius

75 S-1
Piriformis

75 S-1
Piriformis

To Strengthen

K 10 — CX 3
SECOND
LV 1 — CX 9
FIRST

To Weaken

K 10 — CX 3
SECOND
SP 3 — CX 7
CX 7
FIRST

Circulation-Sex Meridian Function 7-9 PM (FIRE Element)
Please note: Triple Warmer and Circulation Sex are related to the Fire element. Refer to the Fire element metaphors preceding Heart and Small Intestine on page 111.

The many functions of the Circulation/Sex Meridian are intimately associated with the hormones and chemical messengers related to all reproduction whether it be appropriate balance in cell production or sexual procreation. It has to do with the nourishment of new cells and the preparation for cell reproduction. It involves the menstruation cycles, ovarian and uterine functions and prostate and testicular functions. This includes the pleasures of sexual love. It also has to do with passing on genetic, cultural, and personal heritage. The Circulation/Sex Meridian is sometimes also called the Pericardium Meridian and relates to the muscular function of the heart and blood vessels, that which keeps the beat steady and appropriate for the external and internal environments.

Do you feel balanced regarding reproduction and sex? What are you doing to see that your legacy will be passed on in your family, work, play, spiritual community? Do you feel that you have sufficient circulation of blood, warmth, nutrition or sexual energy?

Muscles Associated with the Circulation -Sex Meridian:

Muscle: GLUTEUS MEDIUS-
The Gluteus Medius is used to pull the thigh out and rotate the leg. If this muscle is weak, there may be a corresponding high shoulder or hip. There may be a tendency to limp, or the legs may bow out. The test motion involves holding the legs apart.

Feel this muscle at the side and back of the pelvis. It contracts when you lift your foot off the floor to prevent tripping over little things and when you raise your leg to the side.

Circulation-Sex - Gluteus Medius

Test: Position straight leg out to the side with no rotation. Brace on the opposite leg. Pressure is on the ankle to bring it towards the midline. If standing, balance against a wall or a chair.

What little things are you tripping over or bumping into? Do you have any difficulty holding your legs open, literally or figuratively? Are you making mountains out of mole hills, or making mountains into mole hills?

Muscle: ADDUCTORS-
The adductors hold the thigh in, flexing it and rotating it inward. Weakness can make the pelvis tilt down. These muscles are essential to horseback riders. Strain from remaining in the saddles can result in weakness in the adductors and the bow legged posture characteristic of cowboys. The muscle test involves holding the legs together.

Feel these inner thigh muscles contracting when you hold your knees and ankles together to pull your inner thigh close together.

Test: With the feet together and the opposite leg stabilized, pressure is against the inside of the ankle to pull the leg away to the side. If standing, balance against a wall or a chair.

What personally private matters are you protecting? Do you need to share some of these issues, or do you need to keep more things private? Do you have any difficulty holding your legs together, figuratively or literally? Do you feel that you have protected yourself or others enough regarding sexual matters? If you think of your life or current goal as a horse to ride, are you comfortable in the saddle, or saddle sore?

Circulation-Sex - Adductors

Muscle: PIRIFORMIS-
This hip muscle is very important in posture, especially in the position of the sacrum. Weakness on one side can allow the sacrum to twist, resulting in a "knock kneed" posture. The Piriformis is located right next to the sciatic nerve, which is the longest, largest nerve in the body. Sometimes imbalance in this muscles is associated with pain in the low back and down the back of the thigh and leg. When seated, if you find it hard to lift a foot onto the opposite knee, it is a good indication of piriformis inhibition.

Feel this muscle deep inside the pelvis when you have the knee bent at ninety degrees and turned inward.

Test: With knee and hip bent at right angles, the foot brought across the opposite leg as far as possible, heel higher than the knee. Pressure is against the inside of the ankle to bring the foot out to the side while stabilizing the knee. Alternative standing test: Create a right angle at the knee and fully rotate the lower leg medially. Knees should be adjacent to each other. Stabilize the knee on the side of the test. Pressure is against the inside of the lower leg to rotate the leg laterally.

Do you feel knock kneed, or clumsy, literally or figuratively? Is there some small, subtle, or deep issue irritating your nerves or causing you pain, literally or figuratively?

Muscle: GLUTEUS MAXIMUS-
This is considered the strongest muscle and when it is imbalanced, it can have far reaching effects because of the loss of stability in the pelvis. It is frequently associated with misalignment in the neck and an imbalanced position of the head. The motion of the test suggests kicking behind you.

Feel this muscle contract and give shape to your buttocks when moving the thigh posterior to the body, especially with the knee bent at ninety degrees, to eliminate most of the hamstrings action.

Test: Bend the leg 90° and extend the thigh back as far as possible and stabilize at the front of the hip. Pressure is at the back of the knee to bring the thigh forward. Alternatively, stabilize the knee and press at the back of the heel to bring the lower leg down and out. This is a short range of movement only as the knee is not usually pushed in this direction.

Are you adequately utilizing your gross power to maintain overall stability? Are you relying too much on raw strength, when subtleties are called for? Are your sexual urges giving you a pain in the neck OR is your "head" (thinking) interfering with your fulfillment of your physical/survival/procreative needs?

Circulation-Sex - Gluteus Maximus

Testimonials

Touch for Health empowers people to participate in their own creation of wellness, and not rely solely on treatment

A magnificently integrated system of healing utilizing a combination of Eastern and Western disciplines that will benefit my patients through increased health and awareness; a system in which patients can learn self care and allow me to live up to the definition of "doctor as teacher."

TFH provides me with valuable assessment and treatment skills that should make referrals soar. My patients mentioned that they had taken Touch for Health and were very excited about my taking this class!
> —Cheryl Fuller DC

Patients will be able to help themselves as well as their friends and family. I've learned ways of transferring my knowledge to my patients in a much simpler way.
> —Taisuke Jo, DC

I'm glad to have a set prototype system to test and strengthen the body with. I'm excited to practice this work on my friends and family along with my other healing work. I like the wholistic approach. It makes sense to be working equally with emotions, past experiences, sounds, smells, on and on. TFH is clear and direct, honest and whole.
> —Vayya Cain

TRIPLE-WARMER: 9-11 PM

Teres Minor: Iodine
Sartorius, Gracilis, Gastroc., Soleus: C

Triple Warmer Reference

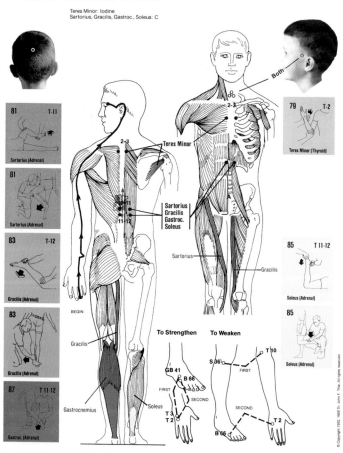

To Strengthen
To Weaken

Triple Warmer Meridian Function 9-11 PM (FIRE Element)

Please note: Triple Warmer and Circulation- Sex are related to the Fire element. Refer to the Fire element metaphors preceding Heart and Small Intestine on page 111.

The Triple Warmer is a somewhat mysterious Meridian in that it is said to have Organ Function in the Chinese energy system, yet it is not associated with a specific organ. It is said to have function, but no form, or it is alternatively defined as having its functions through the interactions of three different groups of organs found in the thoracic, upper and lower abdominal areas. The functions of the Triple Warmer take the form of three "heats", the heat of metabolism and maintaining body heat, the heat of the "fight or flight" and the heat of life passions.

Triple Warmer Function is associated with various interactions of gland secretions involved in our various human passions. The adrenal glands function in concert with other hormonal glands, particularly in fighting or running away in a moment of crisis, or recovery from injury, illness, malfunction and generalized stress. Four of the muscles that are related to this meridian function are muscles involved in running, pushing off, or getting on your toes, all essential fight or flight/passion muscles. The pituitary gland works in concert with other endocrine glands that have functions related the heat of life passions, procreative activity and sexual pleasure, life and death circumstances, causes worth suffering and dying for, etc

What gets you hot, physically, mentally, spiritually or emotionally? What are you running from? What are you fighting? Do you feel that your life is one of constant fight or flight? Are you always on the run? What are you willing to suffer or even to die for? Do you feel that you have the fire, the passion, to reach your goals, or die trying?

Muscles Associated with the Triple Warmer Meridian

Muscle: TERES MINOR-
This shoulder muscle rotates the arm and forearm and can be involved in wrist and elbow problems. With weakness on one side, the hands will be turned differently when the arms are allowed to hang down to the side. The action of the muscle test suggests opening the arms or gathering things in. This muscle is associated with the 3 "heats" of the triple warmer meridian, particularly the heat of metabolism associated with thyroid function. The thyroid function involves the balance of metabolism in breaking down or regenerating tissues as well as maintaining body temperature and fat content.

Feel this small muscle between the lower tip of the shoulder blade and the back of the humerus head/top of the arm, when the forearm is bent about 100 degrees at the elbow and the hand is open facing away from the body and rotated externally.

Test: Bend the elbow to 90° and hold it about a fist width to the side of the body, thumb towards shoulder. Turn forearm out as far as possible. Brace at the elbow on the side of the test. Pressure is against the forearm, just above the back of the wrist to push the forearm across the chest.

What do you need to be more or less open about? Do you need to open your arms to receive or are you trying to take in too much? Are you having difficulty assimilating or making efficient use of the nourishment in your life, literally or figuratively? Do you feel that you run too hot or too cold, too fat or too lean?

Muscle: SARTORIUS-
This is the longest muscle in the body. It serves to flex the leg and thigh and turn the thigh sideways and to flex the pelvis and/or twist the hips. It has been referred to as the "tailor's muscle" as it brings one

Triple Warmar - Teres Minor, Sartorius

leg over the opposite knee to create a lap for working on a piece of clothing. This muscle is associated with the 3 "heats" of the Triple Warmer Meridian, particularly the hormonal heats of "fight or flight" or sexual passion of the pituitary gland. The pituitary gland works in concert with other endocrine glands that have functions related the heat of life passions, procreative needs, life and death circumstances, causes worth suffering and dying for, etc.

Feel this long muscle from the outermost edge of the top of the hip bones across the thigh to the inner portion of the shin bone just below the knee when you are crossing your foot to the opposite knee and lowering the same knee as far as possible.

Test: With the leg turned out, knee slightly bent, and the foot brought over the other leg, just below the knee. Pressure is against the ankle and the top of the knee to bring the foot out and straighten the leg.

Do you feel like you have the strength or the passion to meet the challenges in your work/life, to create or to procreate? Do you feel like you have strength or passion to "go the distance", or to give your all, literally or figuratively? What gets you hot, physically, emotionally, mentally, spiritually, etc.?

Muscle: GRACILIS-

This muscle of the inner thigh works in conjunction with the sartorius and hamstrings in bending the knee. Weakness in this muscle makes it difficult to bend the knee without also flexing the hip, and can contribute to a "knock kneed" posture. This muscle is associated with the 3 "heats" of the Triple Warmer Meridian, particularly the heat of passion in all aspects of living associated with the pituitary gland. The pituitary gland works in concert with other endocrine glands that have functions related the heat of life passions, procreative needs, life and death circumstances, causes worth suffering/dying for.

Feel this inner muscle contracting from the pubic bone down the inside of the thigh to just below the knee, when you put one foot over the top of the opposite foot and bring your thighs together.

Test: With the knee bent about 45 degrees, hold the knee steady, pressure is against the inside of the ankle to push the foot out to the side. Alternate test: fully rotate the leg and foot medially. Pressure is on the inside of the lower leg to move the leg to the side.

Do you feel clumsy when you are passionate about different aspects of your life? Are you shy about displaying your passions, or do your erupting passions get out of your control? What gets you hot, physically, emotionally, mentally, spiritually, etc.?

Muscle: SOLEUS-
This muscle works synergistically with the Gastrocnemius and the Plantaris, having in common the Achilles tendon and the Triceps Surae, the tendenous attachment above the knee of all three of these muscles, to flex the foot and the calf, steadying the foot. Weakness in this muscle may cause a tendency to lean or fall forward. This muscle is associated with the 3 "heats" of the Triple Warmer Meridian, particularly the adrenal hormonal heat related to fight or flight. The adrenal glands function in concert with other hormonal glands, particularly in fighting or running away in a moment of crisis, recovery from injury, illness, malfunction and generalized stress.

Feel this deep calf muscle contract when you are pushing with your toes in a plantar flexion position- (pointing your toes away from you), with your knee bent at approximately ninety degrees.

Test: With the knee bent 90 degrees toes pointed, heel flexed toward the calf, Pressure is against the heel and the sole of the foot to straighten the foot. Alternate test: With the knee bent at a 90° angle, and the toes pointed, brace knee. Pressure is against the heel to straighten the leg.

Do you have difficulty determining when to stand your ground and fight or when to retreat? Do you find that you are overly aggressive, or fearful, in non-crisis situations, or do you fail to "rise to the occasion" when there is a genuine crisis? Do you feel that your life is one never-ending crisis, or an endless series of crises?

Muscle: GASTROCNEMIUS-

This muscle works synergistically with the Soleus and the Plantaris, having in common the Achilles tendon the Triceps Surae, the tendenous attachment above the knee of all three of these muscles to flex the foot and the calf, steadying the foot. Weakness can cause hyperextension of the knee, inability to rise up on the toes, or difficulty in bending the knees. This muscle is associated with the 3 "heats" of the Triple Warmer Meridian, particularly the adrenal hormonal heat related to the mechanism of fight or flight. The adrenal glands function in concert with other hormonal glands, particularly in fighting or running away in a moment of crisis, recovery from injury, illness, malfunction and generalized stress.

Feel this superficial calf muscle starting behind the knee and ending at the common tendon of the heel, when the toes are pointed away from the knee, while the knee is slightly bent. A stronger contraction can be felt if the toes are pushing against the ground or an object.

Test: With leg straight and toes pointed, pressure is at the ball of the foot to straighten. Alternative test: Bend the knee slightly, point the toes and brace the knee. Pressure is on the heel to straighten the leg.

What are you running to or from? Do you have difficulty determining when to stand your ground and fight or when to retreat? Do you find that you are overly aggressive, or fearful, in non-crisis situations, or do you fail to "rise to the occasion" when there is a genuine crisis? Do you feel that your life is one never-ending crisis, or an endless series of crises?

Triple Warmar Gastrocnemius

The Wood Element

Gall Bladder And Liver Meridians

The **Wood Element** metaphor is symbolized by green growing things. The Wood Element is fed by and springs from the water element, Which can be thought of in terms of water feeding the roots of a tree, or even the original birth of life in the water element of the ocean. The Wood Element provides fuel for the Fire Element, nourishing its growth. The Wood Element controls the Earth Element by putting roots into the ground and holding it in place. The Wood Element is controlled by the Metal Element, which chops it and can destroy or transform it.

How does the image of Green growing things relate to your life and your goals? Do you have enough roots to sustain your growth, and enough fuel to sustain your passions? Do you have enough structure in your growth so that you can achieve your purposes, or do you need to allow yourself more freedom in your growth to be fulfilled?

The **Color** metaphor associated with the Wood Element is **Green**. We might associate this with the green of new buds on a plant, and with all new birth and growth.

What does the color Green mean to you in your life, related to your current life goals? Is there enough new growth in your life, or are you giving birth to more new ideas, projects, etc. than can be sustained?

The **Season** metaphor for the Wood Element is **Spring**. This is the time of rebirth after the dying and dormancy of winter, the time to come out of hibernation, and look for new beginnings. It is time for planting seeds and developing new ideas.

What does Spring symbolize to you in your life? What in your life

needs to be revived, renewed, or reborn? What seeds do you need to plant now so that you will have a bountiful harvest in the future?

The **Climate** The climate metaphor for the Wood Element is **Wind**. The wind is mysterious and represents the unknown. We do not know when it will come or from where. Wind can be refreshing, helping us to renew our efforts, or it can be harsh and destructive, blowing us into chaos. Wind represents grace, the undeserved favor, but it can also be an undeserved injury, or one that is no one's fault.

What might Wind symbolize in your life? Do you need "a breath of fresh air, a Spring Cleaning or are you being blown away by uncertainty and change?

The **Odor** associated with the Wood Element is **Rancid**, the smell of spoiled oil, or fat. We might visualize the leftover oils, leftover supplies, which have lasted the winter but now need to be replaced. This could also relate to any of the hormones that relate to all of the emotions and their regulation. We might think of the fats and oils of the body smoothing our movements, or being stagnated and rancid from lack of activity and circulation.

What does a Rancid smell mean in your life? What do you need to let go of that was useful, but is now Rancid? Do you feel stagnant physically, emotionally, mentally or spiritually? How can you get things moving smoothly?

The **Taste** associated with the Wood Element is **Sour**. The Sour flavor can relate to good things that have gone bad, such as spoiled milk, or things that are overpowering in concentration, but delicious when sufficiently balanced or diluted, such as lemonade. It may be time to throw out the old to make room for the new, or it may be time to transform your attitude or your resources to have a positive outcome. Sour might relate to bad attitude- grouchy, grumpy.

What does the Sour flavor represent in your life or related to your goal? Has something that was good gone bad? Do you need to transform sour lemons into lemonade?

The **Emotion** associated with the Wood Element is **Anger**. Anger often masks other feelings such as grief or fear. We may move into Anger to protect old wounds or as a reaction to fear of some danger, or perceived attack or indignity, whether physical, emotional or otherwise. If we find we habitually react in anger, it helps to recognize our grief and fears, and evaluate the appropriate object of anger and the appropriate action to take. Anger can lead to joy when we can be conscious of its source and then feed the fire for our passions for appropriate action, change or growth.

What does Anger mean in your life, or in relation to your goals? Are you angry with yourself or someone else? Does your anger seem to be directed at the appropriate person or thing? Do you need to awaken your outrage, or passions in general, in order grow and reach your goals?

The Sound associated with the Wood Element is Shouting. Shouting may be associated particularly with anger, but it can express any strong feeling. You can shout with joy, pleasure, compassion, grief, fear, awe, etc. Shouting may relate to giving full voice to your emotions, your message or your story. It may be proclaiming joy or determination, crying out in shock or surprise, warning of danger, screaming in fear, bellowing in pain, or yelling encouragement, praise or celebration, etc. Our energy may be imbalanced if we are blocked and unable to express these sounds or express them inappropriately. Shouting can be very empowering and a great release, but if we habitually shout, we may need to assess whether our motivations and the circumstances warrant this behavior.

What does Shouting represent in your life? Are you able to express yourself and give full voice to your feelings and ideas? Are you

"blowing a lot of hot air" out of self-importance, fear or insecurity? What do you need to shout about, or whom do you need to shout at to reach your goals?

The Wood Element is said to **Fortify the Ligaments**. The Ligaments might represent the "safety chains" for the muscles, so that if a muscle fails to function, the ligaments still hold us together. The Ligaments might represent secondary or back-up systems that prevent malfunction and mistakes in primary systems from resulting major damage.

Are you taking proper precautions for the risks in your life, or do you need to "push the envelope" fulfill your purpose and reach your goals, even if that results in some minor mishaps? Are you habitually running on reserves or secondary systems, risking a total breakdown?

The **Personal Power** metaphor of the Wood Element is **Birth**. We can visualize a child being born into the world, but Birth symbolizes all new beginnings for life, ideas, projects, etc. Birth may relate to the story of our own physical birth and beginnings in life. If we feel out of touch with our own personal power, it may be very important to reconsider our own origins or our original intentions in beginning a certain project. We may be expending energy to achieve things that have little or nothing to do with our dreams and aspirations.

What does Birth symbolize in your life? How does the story of your own birth and early life relate to your life and this goal? Do you need a fresh start? Is there something you need to let out, to give birth to, to express your personal power or are you starting too many new things, birthing more than you can support, nourish, and enjoy?

The **Worldview/Faith** metaphor Wood Element involves the **Formistic Implicit process** model where structure and function are seen to exist separately. Processes and systems are essentially invisible and mysterious. This corresponds to the pre-faith stage of Infancy and the Intuitive stage of Early Childhood. It can be called **Intuitive-Projective Faith**. We begin to distinguish some separateness between the world and ourselves and to make use of speech and symbols to make meaning. We have difficulty seeing cause and effect at this stage and are given to **"magical thinking"**. IMAGINATION, dream and vision imagery is essential for creating meaning at this stage. We see our own perspective as the only one that exists and assume everyone else sees things in exactly the same way that we do. We tend to act on our implicit beliefs without being aware of them. We may tend to speak or act without thinking, sometimes from internal wisdom, sometimes from ignorance. This might manifest as saying the "right thing" without even knowing where the words have come from, or it may result in "putting your foot in your mouth".

Have you assumed that your own perspective is the same as everyone else's, or do you feel that there is only one correct opinion? Do you need to use your intuition, creative vision and dream imagery to find new meanings, or are you dwelling in your own personal dream-world, ignoring cause and effect, assuming that what seems right to you will be accepted by others?

Testimonials

Touch for Health was developed from the holistic chiropractic approach, and reinforces working with whole people, not diseases

My patients will benefit from my realization as a practitioner that the patients' problems are truly multi-faceted and that TFH can facilitate this reality and reach beyond simple bio-mechanical models of chiropractic health care.

—Richard Warner, DC

I like the whole body/person approach to healing. I can get caught up into fixing "parts". TFH has offered me a new way of thinking and the tools to develop the protocol, in my office, of helping the whole patient.

—Norah Teague DC

TFH is extremely beneficial to evaluate a person as a whole being. TFH will be used on a daily basis in my practice. It's easy to learn and I enjoyed the whole experience.

—Jon Petersen, DC

TFH is such comprehensive work that deals with the person through the whole (psycho) spiritual emotional physical aspects of healing. I had no idea you had taken it that far. Through all the testing and corrections today I feel better than I have in weeks!

—Wendy Jacobson DC

GALL BLADDER: 11 PM-1 AM

Vitamin A

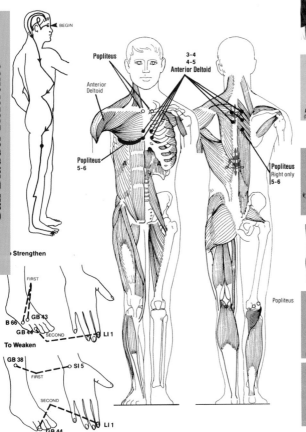

BEGIN

Popliteus

Anterior Deltoid

3-4
4-5
Anterior Deltoid

Popliteus
5-6

Popliteus
Right only
5-6

To Strengthen

FIRST

B 66

GB 43

GB 44

SECOND

LI 1

To Weaken

GB 38

FIRST

SI 5

SECOND

GB 44

LI 1

Popliteus

89 T-4

Anterior Deltoid
(Sitting, Laying, or Standing)

91 T-12

Popliteus
(Sitting, Laying or Standing)

~O~ ~O~

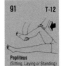

91 T-12

Popliteus

91

Popliteus

Gall Bladder Meridian Function 11 PM to 1 AM

The gall bladder is a small organ that stores and concentrates the bile from the liver, which aids in digestion, particularly of fats. It contracts and releases bile when fats reach the duodenum from the stomach. On a cellular level this same function of maintaining fat metabolism relates to the subtle energy of the Gall Bladder Meridian.

How is your digestion of the heavy parts of your life functioning? Are you diluting your life enough with clear water? Do you remain too concentrated for your own good? Do you need more concentrated juices to deal with the heavy aspects of your life, or are you dealing with too many heavy things?

Muscles Associated with the Gall Bladder Meridian:

Muscle: ANTERIOR DELTOID—
This muscle, along with the coracobrachialis, is used in flexing the shoulder with the elbow bent, as in combing the hair. It is particularly associated with the Gall Bladder Meridian Function of concentrating/releasing bile to aid in digestion of heavy, dense substances such as fats. Inhibition in this muscle is sometimes associated with headaches related to toxicity from dietary indiscretions or eating fatty foods.

Feel this muscle from the front of the shoulder nearest the body to the collar bone when the hand is lifted about twenty degrees from the thigh with the palm down.

Test: Position straight arm slightly less than 45° in front of the body and slightly over the outside of the thigh, palm facing down. Brace on the top of the shoulder on the same side. Pressure is against the forearm to push the arm down.

Do you pay too much or too little attention to the details of grooming, or taking care of yourself? Are you able to "take care"

of your head, or do you do things that result in headache, figuratively or literally? Do you feel that you have too much concentrated bile, or are the heavy aspects of your life overwhelming you? Do you need to dilute or limit the amount of heavy, hard to digest things in your life?

Muscle: POPLITEUS-

This muscle turns the foot and knee in and flexes the leg. When it is inhibited it may increase susceptibility to knee injury. It is sometimes associated with neck pains. In all knee problems this muscle should be carefully evaluated , especially with repeated testing which may indicate a need for prolonged neurolymphatic reflex massage. It is particularly associated with the Gall Bladder Meridian Function of concentrating/releasing bile to aid in digestion of heavy, dense substances such as fats. Inhibition in this muscle is sometimes associated with headaches related to dietary indiscretions .

Feel this small muscle behind the knee when sitting with the leg hanging freely, the foot turned inward, parallel to the ground.

Test: With leg bent and dropped out to the side, stabilize at ankle. Pressure is against the outside of the knee, to twist the lower leg in relation to the thigh. If the popliteus is strong, this torque will be felt in the hip muscles. Alternate test: Create right angles at the ankle and knee and fully rotate the lower leg and foot medially. Brace the heel. Pressure is against the inside of the foot to rotate laterally. If the muscle test is done correctly, the person being tested will feel the muscle's involvement.

What little things are interfering with your movements figuratively and/or literally? Are seemingly small and/or unrelated things resulting in a pain in your neck? Do you feel that you have too much concentrated bile, or are the heavy aspects of your life overwhelming you? Do you need to dilute or limit the amount of heavy, hard to digest things in your life?

Gall Bladder - Popliteus

Testimonials
Touch for Health relieves pain, gets results, and makes you more confident

The balancing that Dr. Thie performed took 80% of my neck pain away. I have needed a review of the course for a long time and feel that if we can teach patients to help themselves at home they will get much more benefit from the treatments as well as make their course of treatments shorter.

—Clayton Neal Meyers DC

Touch for Health really does treat the whole person, not just a symptom picture, named condition, or joint dysfunction. Now I have a tool to help them explore deeper issues that may be impacting their health. Long live TFH!

—Jack Lane DC

I thought that AK is complicated and takes a long time to learn, but today I learned that it can be easy and fun. I really enjoyed the class and learned a lot.

—Mariann Levay DC

The TFH Intensive seminar was fantastic! For me, it resolved old emotional wounds, challenged my mind and significantly improved chronic physical issues. John's teaching method is delightful. One is immersed into the material in a loving spiritual context.

—James Kelly Kindig DC

I have been using TFH and the results are phenomenal!!! I'm already seeing a difference in my practice. Thanks for all the help.

—Serge Gagnon DC

LIVER: 1-3 AM

Liver Reference

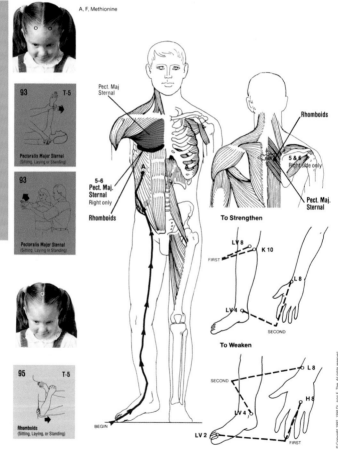

A, F, Methionine

93   T-5

Pectoralis Major Sternal
(Sitting, Laying or Standing)

93

Pectoralis Major Sternal
(Sitting, Laying or Standing)

95   T-5

Rhomboids
(Sitting, Laying, or Standing)

Pect. Maj Sternal

5-6
Pect. Maj.
Sternal
Right only

Rhomboids

Rhomboids

5 & 6
Right side only

Pect. Maj.
Sternal

To Strengthen

LV 8   K 10
FIRST

L 8

LV 4

SECOND

To Weaken

SECOND   L 8

H 8

LV 4

LV 2

FIRST

BEGIN

Liver Meridian Function 1 to 3 AM

The liver has more known functions than any other organ. Each cell has more programmed instructions than the most sophisticated computer program, and the Liver Meridian may activate a large number of the absorption and detoxification instructions. The liver is the largest physical organ and is most active while you sleep. The liver is said to store blood while the body is at rest, and also to exert particular influence over the lower abdomen, and so is considered of central importance in women's menstrual cycle and sexuality. Liver Meridian Function is involved in digestion, metabolism, storage and distribution of nourishment, filtration, detoxification, and immune function.

How are you handling your multiple responsibilities? Are you open to too many things and becoming overwhelmed/toxic, or do you need to absorb more, literally or figuratively? What needs detoxification in your life, what do you need to let go of? What do you need to bring into your life that will be cleansing, purifying or nourishing?

Muscles Associated with the Liver Meridian

Muscle: PECTORALIS MAJOR STERNAL-

This muscle is responsible for moving the arm in, turning and drawing it forward. The test motion suggests opening up, letting go, or throwing your hands up in triumph or surrender, and it is associated with the over 500 primarily absorption and detoxifying functions of the liver.

Feel this muscle of the chest contract between the breastbone and the top of the arm when the extended arm is brought down towards the center of the body with the thumb pointed to the ground.

Liver - Pectoralis Major Sternal

Test: Position the arm straight forward and level with the shoulder, palm turned out, thumb toward the feet. Pressure is on the forearm to push up and back about 45°.

Are you open to too many things and becoming overwhelmed/toxic, or do you need to absorb more, literally or figuratively? What needs detoxification in your life, what do you need to let go of? What do you need to bring into your life that will be cleansing, purifying or nourishing?

Muscle: RHOMBOIDS-
These muscles in the back of the shoulders pull in and turn the shoulder blade. They are used with the levator scapulae and are rarely found weak. They are also associated with the over 500 primarily absorption and detoxifying functions of the liver.

Feel these muscles contract between the shoulder blades and the spine when you bring your shoulder blades together toward the spine and your shoulders up toward the ears.

Test: With the elbow bent and held against the side of the ribs, bring the shoulders up and back, using the rhomboids to bring the shoulder blades closer together. The shoulder is stabilized and pressure is against the inside of the upper arm to pull it away to the side (similar to the levator scapulae test, but without bringing the elbow to the hip.)

What are you uptight about? Are you holding onto toxic emotions, or retaining any other toxic material? Do you need to take a defensive posture?

Liver - Rhomboids

The Metal Element

Lung and Large Intestine Meridians

The **Metal Element metaphor** corresponds to the hardened, condensed materials that form within the earth. The Earth element gives birth to Metal, symbolized by the condensed ores, minerals or salts which form within the earth. Metal in turn gives birth to Water, which is symbolized by the condensation of water on a metal surface. Metal is controlled by Fire, which melts it and can serve to purify it and give it specific form. Metal controls Wood. In the form of a metal blade, Metal can chop wood and transform it for many purposes. The Metal Element may be associated with hardness used to protect yourself, what armor you wear, what tools or weapons you carry, or it may relate to adornment with shining metals.

Do you need a "hard shell", barriers or boundaries to protect you from the demands or aggressions of people in your life, or do you need to open up more, let down your shield or mask to communicate with people? Are you too hard or not hard enough on yourself or others? Are you too focused on adornment and appearances, or do you need to pay some attention to how you represent and communicate your inner richness and potential?

The **Color** metaphor associated with the Metal Element is White. White light is associated with being honorable, honest, trustworthy, etc. It may also relate to the image of a polished metal shining with reflected light.

What does the color white mean to you in your life, related to your current life goals? Do you have enough of the pure light of truth in your life, or have you been deceived by the mere appearance of truth, the brilliance of shiny things?

Metal Element Metaphors

The **Season** metaphor of the Metal Element is **Autumn**, the time of harvest. We can imagine scenes of the last harvest and the storing of foods for the winter, the beauty of the changing colors of leaves before they drop to the ground.

What in your life is in its Autumn phase? Have you been able to harvest the fruits of your labor, or has disaster befallen your crop, or inattention allowed it to spoil?

The **Climate** metaphor of the Metal Element is **Dryness**. We might imagine a desert scene that is generally very dry, but nevertheless teeming with life that has adapted to the dry conditions. Too much dryness will even kill cactus, which normally thrives in the hot, dry weather, but too much moisture, especially all of a sudden, can result in flooding and wholesale uprooting, or perhaps root rot from too much damp.

What might Dryness symbolize in your life? Do you need a little more moisture for lubrication and growth or are you too damp or even flooded? Do you need to concentrate and store that which nourishes you (the life giving waters), or do you need a chance to "dry out"?

The **Odor** metaphor for the Metal Element is **Rotten**. We might imagine something that is over ripe, and beginning to decompose such as fallen leaves or fruit that has fallen unharvested. It may be that an aspect of your life is being affected by immoral or corrupt behavior or influences. Perhaps, "Something is rotten in Denmark".

What is rotten in your life? Are you simply aware of the aroma of the necessary dying of some things so that other things can grow, or have you allowed good and valuable things to become corrupt, to rot, and to go to waste?

The **Taste** metaphor for the Metal Element is **Pungent**. Imagine

Metal Element Metaphors

something that is very spicy, sharply affecting the organs of taste, even burning, or stinging. Pungent or spicy can be a metaphor for anything that is appealing, stimulating, exciting, or tantalizing in your life.

Is there enough sharpness and spice in your life or is it too hot, painful or dangerous? Do you need to "spice things up" to reach your goal, or would you be more successful if you took a more bland approach?

The **Emotion** metaphor of the Metal Element is **Grief**. You might picture yourself standing by a tombstone, suffering pain due to loss or regret. You may have made an error, lost an opportunity, lost a loved one or suffered some mishap, hardship, or a complete disaster. In our modern western culture, grieving has largely been lost as a cultural concept. We are told "Get over it", to "move on with life," etc. This can lead to a chronic failure to attach value to anyone or anything in our lives and a chronic callousness, hardness or indifference. Many times, in order to move on, we need to be able to recognize the damage and loss that we have suffered, express the pain, and realistically assess what we can "get over" and what we must accept as an ongoing aspect of our lives.

What has to be given up, let go, or let die so that you can reach your goals? What have you lost, or has hurt you, that you need to recognize and grieve over?

The **Sound** metaphor of the Metal Element is **Weeping**. We might picture tears running down the face of a person. These tears might be shed in sadness, fear or grief, but we can also cry for Joy or in awe, sympathy, empathy, compassion, or even anger. Allowing tears to flow when appropriate is very healthy and helpful for our balance and wholeness. If we are too hardened to cry, this can block our life energy. If someone says, "I never cry" it may indicate unhealed wounds or an ossified siege mentality. There are times when we must "keep a stiff upper lip" to survive or get through a situation, but to deny the flow of tears completely can be toxic.

How does the sound of weeping relate to your current goals? Do you hold in too much weeping or are you prone to crying a lot or when it's not appropriate?

The Metal Element is said to **Fortify the Skin and Hair**. This might relate to personal grooming or attention to personal appearance. How you represent yourself as well as how you take care of yourself. The skin is a major organ and is very important for detoxification. The skin actually "breathes". Our skin and hair can act as our "armor" or as "antennae". We can retreat defensively within our shell, or attune ourselves to all of the vibrations we can sense with the skin and hair.

Do you take personal responsibility for your own hygiene and is that reflected in your appearance? Do you take enough, or too much responsibility for how others see you, or perceive you? Are you "thin skinned" or "thick skinned"?

The **Personal Power** metaphor for the Metal Element is **Balance**. You might imagine a set of scales as a symbol of balance, or the symbol of the yin and yang.

How do you need to be more balanced to have more personal power and achieve your goals? What aspects of your life are out of balance and decreasing your power in your own experience.

The **Faith/Worldview** metaphor of the Metal Element relates to Young Adulthood. In this phase all of the "parts" of our life are integrated to form a whole system. All structures and functions reflect organization of the interactive relationships. This is the phase of **Responsible Faith or Individuative-Reflective belief**. At this stage we begin to assume personal responsibility for our own personal lifestyle, beliefs, and attitudes. We work to construct an individual, rational, functional worldview. Symbols are considered as conceptual/metaphorical, rather than having singular, literal, fixed meaning. Paradoxes, polarities, and complexity are a challenge at this stage as we balance our personal priorities and seek to distinguish relative and absolute truths.

Do you feel that you can take personal responsibility for your beliefs and your actions, or do you feel that your life is shaped by the roles you play for others and the meaning you have in the life of others? Are you being too literal in your beliefs, or perhaps letting your sense of responsibility slip according to circumstances.

Metal Element Metaphors

Lung Reference

LUNG: 3-5 AM

C. Water

101	T 3-4

Deltoids
(Sitting, Laying, or Standing)

97	T 3-4

Ant. Serratus
(Sitting, Laying, or Standing)

99	T-2

Coracobrachialis
(Sitting, Laying, or Standing)

103	T 12

Diaphragm
(Sitting, Laying, or Standing)

103	

Diaphragm
(Sitting, Laying, or Standing)

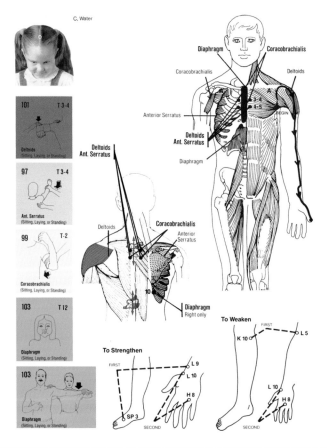

Diaphragm   Coracobrachialis

Coracobrachialis

Deltoids

Anterior Serratus

BEGIN

Deltoids
Ant. Serratus

Diaphragm

Deltoids
Ant. Serratus

Deltoids

Coracobrachialis

Anterior
Serratus

Diaphragm
Right only

To Strengthen

FIRST

L 9

L 10

H 8

SP 3

SECOND

To Weaken

FIRST

K 10   L 5

L 10

H 8

SECOND

Lung Meridian Function 3 to 5 AM

While we may not go without water for much more than a few days, or without food for more than a week or two, we usually can't last without air for more than about three minutes. The lungs are the chief organs of respiration and exchange of gases, mainly oxygen and carbon dioxide, serving both as a primary and essential source of life energy as well as an important channel of elimination. The lungs also supply the air for speaking and making other vocal sounds. In addition to drawing in air (oxygen), the Lung Meridian Function is said to draw in or release Chi, and regulate the status of chi in the whole Soul.

Can you breath/speak easily? Do you have a free flow of fresh air and/or inspiration to nourish the various functions of your life, or are you feeling constricted, inhibited in speaking, literally or figuratively? What do you need to lift up in your life? Are you giving too much or too little praise? Do you need to shout, cheer, or even cough something up?

Muscles Associated with the Lung Meridian

Muscle: ANTERIOR SERRATUS-

This large strong muscle draws the shoulder forward and raises the ribs. Weakness will make it difficult to push things forward with the arms straight. Chronic weakness of this muscle lets the shoulder blade pull away from the posterior chest. It is a muscle that needs to be functioning fully for ideal breathing and activities that require good breath control, and it is associated with Lung Meridian Function. Bilateral weakness is sometimes associated with neck pain, and rotating the head and neck may loosen and relieve this pain.

Feel this muscle contract on the side of the chest when you hold your arm in front of you and then reach forward with power as if you were going to punch.

Test: Position the straight arm in front and slightly higher than the shoulder, thumb pointed up, fingers extended. Hold the tip of the shoulder blade on the same side to ensure it remains stable. Pressure is against the forearm to bring the arm toward the feet.

Do you need to exert your power to reach your goal? Do you need to push, or punch, or are you pushing so hard that you're giving yourself a pain in the neck, or even forgetting to breath, literally or figuratively? Have you lost your voice literally or figuratively?

Muscle: CORACOBRACHIALIS-

This small shoulder muscle works with the anterior deltoid in straitening the arm when it is held over the head and in flexing the shoulder with the elbow bent, as in combing the hair. It can be associated with a lot of shoulder pain and suffering when it is not functioning properly. As with all muscle testing in the Touch for Health System, if there is pain when attempting to feel the muscle in the testing position, consider the muscle inhibited (in need of reflex activity for restoration of full function). The test motion suggests a gesture associated with shouting, cheering, or maybe even coughing, and it is associated with Lung Meridian Function.

Feel this small muscle under the Deltoid between the front of the arm and the anterior portion of the shoulder blade when raising you hand as if to comb your hair, put on make-up or shave.

Test: With elbow bent as far as possible, palm toward the shoulder and the arm 45 degrees up and 45 forward, pressure is against the biceps in the middle of the upper arm to push the arm back and toward the body.

Following the metaphor of combing the hair or grooming, do you pay too much or too little attention to the details of grooming, or taking care of yourself? Is it easy to "take care" of yourself, or is it painful to care for yourself, literally or figuratively? Do you

need to shout, cheer, or even cough something up? Have you lost your voice literally or figuratively?

Muscle: DELTOIDS-
This muscle draws the arm up and away from the body, lifting the elbow. It may be involved in any shoulder problem and it is associated with Lung Meridian Function. Weakness in this muscle may make it difficult to raise the arm. It has bursae under it, between it and the bone, which can become inflamed and even have calcium deposits in these water sacs. It is important to remember that pain on movement to feel the muscle should be considered the same as weakness and utilize the reflexes for balancing and the challenging procedures.

Feel this strong muscle at the top of the shoulder when you raise the arm from the side of the body toward the head.

Test: With the arm held out to the side, elbow level with the shoulder and bent 90 degrees. Pressure is just above the elbow to push it down to the side of the body.

What do you need to lift up in your life? Are you giving too much or too little praise? Do you need to lift up your arms and shout alleluia? Are you getting enough inspiration, or do you feel stale?

Muscle: DIAPHRAGM-
This muscle separates the chest cavity from the abdominal cavity. It is the chief muscle used in breathing and it is associated with Lung Meridian Function. It is essential to ease in speaking and singing. When the diaphragm is not functioning properly, it is associated with unusual symptoms because of the many neurological centers near it, as well as the holes for the esophagus, aorta, vena cava (large blood vessels), the vagus nerves and the large lymphatic vessel. When functioning ideally, the diaphragm assists in the function of these systems.

Feel this dome shaped muscle between the spine the lower ribs and breast bone. It separates the chest cavity from the abdominal cavity. When you breathe in, it lowers and pushes the abdominal contents down. When you breathe out, it rises and helps you empty your lungs.

Test: Circuit locate the diaphragm. Place two fingers over the diaphragm (at the tip of the breast bone- the xiphoid process) and test any previously strong indicator muscle to see if it becomes inhibited. You can also test to each side of the xiphoid process. Additional Test: Take a deep breath and hold it in. Time should be at least 40 seconds. After working the reflexes, time may increase by 1/3 to 1/2.

Can you breathe easily? Do you have a free flow of fresh air and/or inspiration to nourish the various functions of your life, or are you feeling constricted, literally or figuratively? Are you able to speak comfortably, is speaking taxing or have you lost your voice, literally or figuratively? Do you need to sing?

Lung - Diaphragm

Testimonials

The Touch for Health Intensive Seminar with Dr. John F. Thie is an inspiring, transforming experience

In the TFH intensive seminar I learned muscle testing, all the different ways of balancing, listening/ communication/ interviewing skills, keeping "wholeness of the soul" when discussing health care. I feel more confident as a person and practitioner. I have already changed my attitude and I'm even driving my car differently. Watching others in class open up and seeing positive changes is amazing. The training is so hands on and experiential from both sides (giving & receiving balances) that the material not only gets into the head but into the body. TFH has supplied us with the instruction booklet which unlocks many secret keys in the body. I feel the TFH intensive seminar gave me more practical tools to balance a person than I got out of 3 years of oriental medical school. Thank you,
— Hoberleigh Phreigh

The elimination in my chronic low back pain and drastic improvement of my vision are priceless!
— Rudy Hunter

TFH has inspired me to be more aware and to take care of myself and to help other people to be balanced, to live a healthy, productive, peaceful life. The training is top quality, enjoyable, energizing, understandable, empowering, life-changing. I learned the muscle tests so well by seeing, doing, experiencing and being balanced each day and discovering about my life, what blocks my energy & vitality!! I am confident I have it down.
— Barbara Trask

Large Intestine Reference

LARGE INTESTINE: 5-7 AM

Fascia Lata: Iron, B, Lactobacillus
Hamstrings: E
Quadratus Lumborum: E, A, C

105   L-2
Fascia Lata

105
Fascia Lata

109   L 4-5
Quadratus Lumborum

109
Quadratus Lumborum

Fascia Lata
Hamstrings

L 5

BEGIN

Hamstrings

Quadratus
Lumborum

Fascia Lata
Both sides

To Strengthen

S 36 — LI 11

FIRST

SI 5 — LI 5

SECOND

To Weaken

LI 5
SI 5 — SECOND

FIRST

SI 5

B 66

LI 2

107   L 4-5
Hamstrings

107
Hamstrings

Large Intestine Meridian Function 5 to 7 AM

The Large Intestine Function is to absorb the last useful products of digestion and store the waste materials until they can be eliminated. Approximately 80% of the material entering the large intestines is absorbed, but it is mostly water. The Large Intestine Meridian Function is very important in the metabolism of water, extracting water from waste material and either reabsorbing it or sending it on to the bladder, and passing waste material as stool. It is also crucial in eliminating waste materials, as imbalance in the Large Intestine Function may result in physical, mental, emotional or spiritual toxicity.

Do you retain things you can no longer use in your life or are you letting too much go out of your life? What are you hanging onto that is toxic, literally or figuratively?

Muscles Associated with the Large Intestine

Muscle: FASCIA LATA-

This very long muscle has its bulk on the pelvis and then a very thin band of tissue runs down the side of the leg to just below the knee. The fascia lata helps flex or bend the thigh, draw away from the body sideways, and keep it turned in. With weakness, the legs may tend to bow, the thigh turning outward. In walking and running it helps to align the planting of the foot. When it is not functioning ideally, the foot is turned outward and the toes are not used in the most effective way to give power to the forward thrust in walking or running. This muscle is particularly associated with the Large Intestine Meridian Function of absorbing the beneficial nutrients before waste products are passed on. Approximately 80% of the material entering the large intestines is absorbed.

Feel this muscle at the top and side of your pelvis and on the side of your leg when you turn your foot inward.

Test: With the leg raised up approximately 45° and slightly to the side, the foot turned in, pressure is against the outside of the ankle to push the leg down and in. Stabilize the opposite hip so that the body doesn't rotate.

Do you feel that you have power and thrust in your walk (or race) of life? Can you open your legs and still retain power/control, or can you hold your legs closed if you want to, literally or figuratively? Do you tend to throw the baby out with the bath water, or you hanging on to material that needs to be let go?

Muscle: HAMSTRINGS-
This very strong muscle on the back of the thigh is very important in running and turning while running. It can be injured if not functioning optimally when running and turning the foot. It flexes and turns the leg sideways when the knee is bent. Inhibition in this muscle is associated with bow-legged or knock-kneed posture, as well as toxicity and headaches. This muscle is particularly associated with the Large Intestine Meridian Function of absorbing the beneficial nutrients before waste products are passed on. Approximately 80% of the material entering the large intestines is absorbed.

Feel this large muscle on the back of your thigh between the pelvis and the knee when you straighten out your leg from a bent position. Like the triceps in the arm it is an eccentric contractor.

Test: With the leg bent slightly less than 90°, stabilize the knee, pressure is against the back of the Achilles' tendon to straighten leg.

Do you feel that you have enough power to move and run, or are you expending too much power, literally or figuratively? Are you able to make changes while in full stride? Has a change/shift while in full motion caused you some strain, injury or discomfort, literally or figuratively? Do you tend to throw the baby out with the bath water, or you hanging on to material that needs to be let go?

Muscle: QUADRATUS LUMBORUM-

This muscle flexes the vertebral column sideways, drawing it toward the hip. It assists the action of the diaphragm in breathing. It is a major stabilizing muscle of the low back. It is a very strong muscle and is very important when any back pain is present. When it isn't functioning properly it can effect the function of the diaphragm, and so can be associated with almost any symptom.

Feel this deep low back muscle contract between the lowest ribs and the top of the pelvis in the back when you tilt yourself to the side without bending forward or backward.

Test: With the person either lying face up or down and using their hands to keep torso stable, take both legs out to one side, stabilize the opposite hip. Pressure is at the outside of the ankle to press both legs toward the mid-line. Lift the legs high enough that the feet will clear the table or floor. Alternative standing test: Lean your hips to one side and your shoulders to the other with the feet together. Place one hand on the extended hip and the other on the opposite shoulder. Pressure with both hands is towards the midline.

Are you functioning in an upright way literally or figuratively? What is giving you a pain in the back? How do you need to give yourself greater stability? Does your work/life/goal require you to bend more than is comfortable, literally or figuratively? Could you benefit from some flexibility and being able to bend like a reed in the wind, yielding, yet strong?

Nutrition

Lately there has been a lot of commotion about good nutrition - vitamins, proteins and health foods. Much new information is coming out all the time, but the basics are clear. Proper nutrition is absolutely essential to good health. The simplest guide is 'eat only whole foods.' If a food is processed or broken down into another form - avoid it. Stay as close to the natural state of the food as is reasonable. The ground rule is always, 'fresh food is best.' Frozen food is usually better than canned, but the goal is to eat a variety of natural foods in their natural state and to eat all the different parts of them. The nutritional suggestions, which are listed with each of the different muscles, are there only as a guide. Most of these things would normally be included in a complete diet. However, if a person for some reason has a particular need or is not getting enough of one of these things, this can show up as a persistent weakness of certain muscles. These nutritional elements seem to help the most when they are taken in their natural form as food and chewed thoroughly, rather than in a highly concentrated pill or synthetic vitamin. Chewing does more than chop the food into smaller pieces and mix the saliva with the food, beginning the first stage of digestion and the breakdown of the food into then different elements and fuels. The chemical reactions that take place in the mouth with the saliva are enough to trigger the brain to call out all the necessary action from the rest of the body which will be required to process the food. This seems to be a very important but little-known function of the mouth, which is evidently a very sensitive mechanism .If a particular weakness exists, it may be caused by a nutritional deficiency normally associated with that particular muscle. After the muscle has been tested and before any other treatment has been used, have the person chew for a few moments on one of the suggested foods containing a high level of that particular nutrient. If the body seems to need that element, the muscle will immediately respond, can be tested and will show an improvement in strength. This reaction is almost instantaneous, once the food has mixed with the saliva and has been in the mouth

Food Testing Basics:
BIOGENIC - foods and substances that raise our energy, do not take too much energy to digest, and leave little residue for the body to eliminate. A locked muscle will stay locked, or an unlocked muscle will lock when testing foods and substances that are biogenic. (Use the Sensitivity Mode to get more information)
BIOSTATIC - foods and substances that have a neutral effect on us. A muscle test will remain unaffected when testing foods and substances that are biostatic. (If the muscle test remained locked, use the Sensitivity Mode to get more information)
BIOCIDIC - foods and substances that downgrade our energy, take an extra amount of energy to digest, and leave toxic waste for the body to eliminate. A locked muscle will unlock and an unlocked muscle will remain unlocked when testing foods and substances that are biocidic. (There is no need to use the Sensitivity Mode in this situation).

Food Testing (with C1)
In Touch For Health, muscle testing has enabled us to 'individualize' our nutrition. What is said to be 'good food' may NOT be good for an individual person right now. We can use muscle testing to help us develop our awareness of our nutritional requirements and avoid foods (substances) that are not helpful. It should be clearly remembered that the person being tested should choose their preferred method of testing, being aware that some substances can have an adverse reaction on some people. The following system improves the accuracy of food testing without adding much to the time.

1. Do the usual pre-checks and use an IM to circuit locate C1. If this is clear, go to Method A or B
2. If the circuit locating indicates, clear in the following way:
Bilaterally test Supraspinatus. Correct using SR's, NL's, NV's, etc.
3. Repeat step one. If C1 does not clear, further testing may be unreliable. Use the indicator muscles for each meridian instead.

Evaluation Method A (using a locked Indicator Muscle):

1. Do usual pre-checks and using a locked Indicator Muscle, ask the person to hold the food (chewing it some, ideally) in the mouth and Retest the IM:
Locked = Probably Biostatic or Biogenic - go to step 2
Unlocked = Biocidic - Impairs Balance
(No need to check C1)
2. Have the person circuit locate C1.
3. Retest the probable biogenic / biostatic food/supplement now.

Locked IM = Probably OK to eat (or drink).

Unlocked IM = While there may be some balancing effect, overall it is biocidic.

Evaluation Method B (using an unlocked Indicator Muscle):

1. Do usual pre-checks. Use an unlocked indicator muscle to test and ask the person to hold the food (chewing it some, ideally) in the mouth and Retest the IM:
Locked IM = probably Biogenic - go to step 2
Unlocked IM = biostatic or biocidic
2. Have the person circuit locate C1.
3. Retest the probable biogenic food/supplement now

Locked IM = Probably helpful to eat (or drink)

Unlocked IM = While there may be something in the food that is beneficial, this is probably NOT the form for you to take it in at this time.

BALANCING WITH FOOD

Food causes a reaction in the whole person even before it reaches the stomach. As soon as we see the food, think about it, and especially once we begin to smell the food, the digestive process has begun. This process takes place in parallel on the neurological, chemical, and subtle energy levels. We can tap into this very powerful process and use food as a reflex to balance the energy of the person. Remember, we do not prescribe or treat in Touch for Health, even with food.

1. Do any usual pre-checks, and set a goal.

2. Do a 14 muscle assessment and determine the meridian that would be the appropriate place to start based on the 24 hour cycle or the 5 Element cycles.

3. On the Muscle Reference page, find the foods associated with the meridian, and have the person pick one of the foods that are recommended. Choose only foods that the person knows they do not have a reaction to.

4. While the person chews and holds the food in the mouth, recheck all the previously inhibited muscles. Usually, the muscles are now facilitated.

5. Challenge by swallowing the food and re-testing. You can check the "sensitivity" mode to confirm.

6. Reassess the goal.

Bon appétit!

Balancing with Food

Four Health Roles

When optimizing our health, we need to be aware of our different roles according to our health status. Our goals for our health, and the focus of our activities can be quite different, depending on whether we are healthy, sick, recovering/rehabilitating, or dying.

When healthy, we're aware of our health and energy needs, we are pro-active and take responsibility for the choices that lead to greater vitality and fulfillment. When we consult with a professional, we want to be informed and formulate our own opinion based on our personal knowledge of ourselves together with the advice of experts.

When we are in an emergency situation, we may need to take a more passive role and trust in the decisions of emergency medical personnel. If we are pro-active while we are healthy, we will have people to contact who can be our advocates when we are injured or very sick. In the sick role we may give up the position of first authority as to our best treatment, but we still want to be aware, to the extent possible, of our condition and outlook, and make sure there is some advocacy for treatment/outcomes that are right for us.

When we are recovering/rehabilitating, we may or may not have some ongoing treatment regime, but we again take responsibility for the ongoing choices we make that lead to improvement in quality of life. We may need to accept temporary or ongoing limitations or challenges, but find fulfillment within our current range of function. However, in our culture, we sometimes expend a great deal of energy and resources prolonging life, when our efforts might be better spent focussing on having a good death.

Even in death, there is great potential for quality experiences. There are things that we want to focus on, and things we want to de-emphasize. When in the dying role, we want to let go of heroic measures meant to "save" us, which might prolong "life" yet distract us from our goals. We want to avail ourselves of treatment that will allow us to make the most of the time we have with the ones we love. Balancing our energy with TFH can help our functioning in each of these roles.

Conclusion

Additional Touch for Health Reference Materials

Touch for Health Book   **29.95**
Basic Text describing TFH method & reference photographs of all 42 TFH muscle tests and diagrams of all touch reflex points.

Touch for Health Reference Wall Chart   **35.95**
29 X 43 inches, laminated, color coded. Contains graphic reference to all of the TFH reference points, including thumbnails of muscle tests.

Touch for Health Reference Folio   **23.95**
9 X 12 approx. Same diagrams as Wall Chart in a spiral bound folio.

Touch for Health Reference Pocket Folio   **19.95**
Scaled down version fits your lab-coat, pocket, purse or backpack

Acupuncture Meridian Chart   **18.95**
35 X 23, laminated. Illustration of all the acupuncture points along the 14 major meridian pathways. Meridian balancing/ pain control.

TFH Law of 5 Elements Chart   **24.95**
24 X 32, laminated. Wall Poster for Energy Assessment

Thorson's Introductory Guide to Kinesiology   **11.00**
TFH history and development of different kinesiology systems

TFH 24 hr. Law and 5 Elements Law Booklet   **9.00**
Explains use of Assessment chart, and Acupressure Holding Points

Improve Your Life with TFH, Video   **24.95**
Perfect Complement to TFH Book. Features Dr. John F. Thie.

TFH Video, PAL format   **29.95**

Touch for Health Song, by Garrick   **8.95**
Original music for exercise, cross-crawl. Sets pace for 3 min. dance.

Handy Touch for Health Assessment Chart   **15.00**
11 X 17, laminated. 24 hr./5-Element chart with 111 metaphor questions color coded to the elements/meridians on the back.

TFH Pocketbook *with* 5-Element Metaphors   **19.95**
184 pages. 61/2 X 4 1/4 inches. Full Color throughout, An introduction to Touch for Health and use of the Chinese 5-Elements in the context of TFH energy balancing. Includes all of the TFH Reference Folio pages, muscle-testing, In-depth Goal-Setting, etc.

Please note: Prices are current at press time but subject to change without notice. To verify price, cost of shipping and order, contact:
Devorss & Co • POB 550 • Marina Del Rey, CA • 90294-0550
(800) 843-5743 in USA • (310) 821- 6290 • FAX (310) 821-6290

TFH Materials

Touch for Health Education maintains a website, organizes seminars by Dr. Thie and Matthew Thie, and Publishes Touch for Health books and charts.

TFHE
Touch for Health Education
6162 La Gloria Drive
Malibu, Ca 90265
888-796-4568 within the United States
FAX 310-589-5369 Telephone 213-482-4480
website: www.touch4health.com
e-mail for Dr. Thie: thie@touch4health.com
e-mail for Matthew Thie: thie1@earthlink.net

Contact information

TFHKA
Touch for Health Kinesiology Association of America
P.O.Box 392
New Carlisle OH, 45244-0392
Telephone: 800-466-8342
FAX: 937-845-3909
website: www.tfhka.org
e-mail: Admin@tfhka.org

The TFHKA is a membership organization dedicated to serving TFH instructors and educating the public about the benefits of TFH and the opportunities for instruction. Contact the association for an instructor near you, Instructor Training, Annual Conferences, and other TFH resources and information

The International Kinesiology College carries on the mission of the Touch for Health Foundation, promoting the concepts of Touch for Health, establishing standards for Touch for Health courses and Instructor Training. For information about a TFH kinesiology association worldwide, contact the IKC.

IKC
International Kinesiology College
Sonnenstrasse 15 CH-8331
Auslikon-Zürich
Phone +41 1 950 05 88
Fax +41 1 950 61 87
e-mail info@ikc-info.com
website www.ikc-info.com